HEALING A VILLAGE

I0112750

HEALING A VILLAGE

A PRACTICAL GUIDE TO BUILDING RECOVERY COMMUNITIES

BY MARK LEFEBVRE

FOREWORD BY DEAGLAN MCEACHERN, MAYOR OF PORTSMOUTH

Peter E. Randall Publisher
Portsmouth, NH
2025

© 2025 Mark Lefebvre
All Rights Reserved.

ISBN: 978-1-942155-87-4 print
ISBN: 978-1-942155-88-1 eBook

Library of Congress Control Number 2025900810

Published by
Peter E. Randall Publisher
5 Greenleaf Woods Drive, U102
Portsmouth, NH 03801

Book Design: Tim Holtz
Cover Design: Eric Ott

Printed in the United States of America

To Vivian, Joey & Selena—
For doing for me what I could not do for myself.

CONTENTS

FOREWORD

It has been my privilege to witness firsthand the incredible strides our community has taken in the fight against addiction, and much of that progress is due to the tireless work of Mark Lefebvre and Pinetree Institute. In this book, *Healing a Village: A Practical Guide to Building Recovery Ready Communities*, Mark offers a blueprint for other communities seeking to build coalitions that are both compassionate and effective.

In Portsmouth, we've seen how a trauma-informed, community-driven approach can transform not only the lives of those in recovery but the entire community. By fostering trust, reducing stigma, and coordinating resources, Mark and Pinetree Institute have set a standard for how municipalities can address addiction through partnership, empathy, and evidence-based practices.

Sadly, the need for this work remains as pressing as ever. Despite all the progress we've made, the challenges posed by addiction continue to affect families and communities. This makes the insights in Mark's book all the more vital. His approach doesn't just offer hope; it offers a practical, proven path forward.

What's particularly powerful about this guide is its emphasis on creating a cohesive framework that enables communities to work together, rather than in silos, to address addiction. Mark shows us how collaboration is not just a goal but a necessity for achieving lasting impact. His framework provides the structure needed to unite different stakeholders—whether in healthcare, government, or local organizations—so that together, we can tackle addiction more effectively.

This guide goes beyond theory. It provides real tools and case studies from right here in New Hampshire, showing how coalitions can thrive, even in the face of seemingly insurmountable challenges. From our own Greater Portsmouth Recovery Coalition to the inspiring work across Strafford and York Counties, the lessons in these pages are practical, hard-won, and deeply needed.

Whether you are a government leader, healthcare provider, or community advocate, this book will provide you with the insights you need to bring recovery-ready principles to life in your own community. As Mark's work has shown us, when we build a coalition that centers on dignity and support, we are not just healing individuals—we are healing the entire village.

—Deaglan McEachern, Mayor of the City of Portsmouth

INTRODUCTION

This book is about hope.

On a Thursday morning in August 2012, I was a day away from being discharged from the Behavioral Health Unit at Portsmouth Regional Hospital. I had spent the previous four days in the unit after planning to take my own life following a long history of substance use, alcoholism, and mental illness. My diagnosis was polysubstance use disorder, major depressive disorder, and generalized anxiety disorder. Collectively, these are recognized clinically as co-occurring disorders.

During my stay, I was medically detoxed from alcohol, opioids, narcotic anti-depressants, narcotic anti-anxiety, and narcotic sleep medications. I was under heavy medication to manage my supervised withdrawal from my daily cocktail of prescription pain pills, Lexapro, Xanax, Ambien, cannabis, and of course, alcohol. I was confused. I was scared. Yet here I sat across the table from my wife, Vivian, in the visitors' area of the unit, discussing my discharge options. She too was confused and scared. And she was angry. In addition to being concerned for my health, she was angry at me for the crisis I had bestowed upon her and our family. But in the moment she was angry at the hospital staff for my discharge plan, which was a listing of mental health counselors who specialized in substance-use disorder and a list of local Alcoholics Anonymous (AA) meetings.

I certainly was in no shape to return home and attempt a recovery plan on my own. I needed a long-term residential program that specialized in co-occurring mental health and substance use disorders. I needed round-the-clock observation. I needed psycho-therapy. And in the moment I needed to be pre-qualified for admission to such a facility prior to my discharge, which was scheduled for the following day.

I was eventually admitted to Michael's House in Palm Springs, California, which offered a twenty-eight-day residential program followed by another twenty-eight days of intensive outpatient (IOP) programming. While in the hospital considering my discharge options, I was fortunate to have my wife with me given my mental state. She had learned about Michael's House from a relative whose sister successfully began her journey of recovery there.

In 2012, there were two inpatient treatment centers in New Hampshire: Farnum Center at Eliot Hospital in Manchester, and Granite Recovery Center in Salem. There were no peer recovery community centers in New Hampshire, as peer recovery support was not yet established as an evidence-based recovery program. There was no medication-assisted treatment (MAT) as we know it today. There were perhaps a few men's recovery residences (sober living homes) in New Hampshire, but their locations and occupancy status were a mystery to me and the clinical staff at the hospital.

The aftercare program at Portsmouth Regional Hospital's Behavioral Health Unit did not offer any alternatives for any of these services because in 2012 they did not know about these programs. Or whether they even existed. Vivian had done the research, made the calls, inquired with our insurance provider, and booked my stay at Michael's House. Today I think back to all the former patients who were discharged from Portsmouth Regional Hospital without any place to go, or any means to get there. Upon my discharge I felt hopeless. I had survived my intervention, but I had struggled with detoxing. I was terrified about my future. My situation was not unique. Nor did it tell the entire story.

According to the National Survey on Drug Use and Health (NSDUH), in 2012 (the year I got sober), there were 23.1 million Americans age twelve or older who needed treatment for an illicit drug or alcohol use problem (per DSM IV), yet 20.6 million of these individuals did not receive treatment at a specialty facility in that year.[1] Specialty treatment is defined as hospital inpatient, drug or alcohol rehabilitation facilities, or mental health centers. The six most reported reasons for not receiving treatment were a) not ready to stop using (40.4 percent), b) no health coverage and could not afford cost (34 percent), c) possible negative events on the job (12 percent), d) concern that receiving treatment might cause neighbors/community to have a negative opinion (11.6 percent), e) not knowing where to go for treatment (9.1 percent), and f) had health insurance but it did not cover treatment or cost (7.9 percent). Loosely categorized, the most reported barriers were not ready to stop, lack of insurance coverage, fear of stigma, or not knowing where to go for help.

Jump ahead nine years and the data is equally alarming. According to the US Department of Health and Human Services/Substance Abuse and Mental Health Services Administration (DHHS/SAMHSA), in 2021, 40.7 million Americans age twelve or older who had an illicit drug or alcohol use disorder needed treatment, yet did not receive treatment.[2] The six most reported reasons were a) not being ready to stop using (36.7 percent), b) having no health care and not being able to afford the cost (24.9 percent, c) not knowing where to go for treatment (17.9 percent), d) not finding a program that offered the type of treatment they wanted (15.8 percent), e) thinking they could handle the problem without treatment (15 percent), and f) being concerned that getting treatment might have a negative effect on their job (14.7 percent).

Simply stated, despite all the money that the US government has poured into treatment and recovery over the last decade, today there are more Americans with an SUD who need help than there were almost ten years ago. People still cannot afford to get that help; they don't know where to get the help, and stigma is still a major barrier to entering treatment.

So why is there a need for this book now? In a word, urgency. I was fortunate. My cycle of addiction occurred before fentanyl and its deadly derivatives became readily available and occupied a ubiquitous presence in today's illicit drug supply. According to the *New York Times*, nearly 110,000 Americans died in 2022 of drug overdoses, "representing a plateau after two years of sharp increases."[3] Overdose deaths had climbed by 30 percent in 2020 and 17 percent in 2022, according to the *Times*.

Since the 1970s, the number of drug overdose deaths in the US has climbed every year, with the exception of 2018. The sharp increases in 2020 and 2022 "were driven for the most part by the major changes of fentanyl availability around so many parts of the country," said Dr. Wilson M. Compton, the deputy director of the National Institute on Drug Abuse, which is part of the National Institutes of Health.[4] Other dangerous drugs such as the animal tranquilizer Xylazine are now appearing in the nation's drug supply, causing even more strain on our public health systems.

As of January 11, 2024, my home state of New Hampshire recorded 381 confirmed drug overdose deaths in 2023 with 46 more cases pending toxicology. The 381 confirmed deaths in 2023 represent a decrease of more than 21 percent over 2022.[5] The decrease is largely attributed to the increasing availability of naloxone (sometimes commercially known as Narcan) and the expansion of recovery resources in the Granite State.[6]

The state of Maine saw a decline of 16 percent between 2022 and 2023. In 2022, a record 723 citizens of Maine died of overdoses compared to 607 in 2023. Officials credit the increasing access to life-saving naloxone and the expansion of treatment programs.[7]

Fentanyl is a synthetic opioid that is up to fifty times stronger than heroin and one hundred times stronger than morphine.[8] Recreational users are dying from what the CDC refers to as "fentanyl poisoning," as the user is often unaware of the source of their drug of choice, which may be cocaine, methamphetamine, benzodiazepines, or even edible cannabis. These street drugs may contain deadly levels of fentanyl without the user knowing or intending to use fentanyl. It is nearly impossible to tell if drugs have been laced with fentanyl unless you test your drugs with fentanyl test strips.

Street fentanyl, which is manufactured in Mexico, is plentiful and it is potent. Cartels in Mexico import precursor ingredients from Chinese chemical and pharmaceutical companies. Most fentanyl manufacturing is controlled by the Sinaloa Cartel based in northwestern Mexico and operating worldwide. According to bestselling author Sam Quinones, "The unrelenting supply the cartels create means fentanyl is now everywhere. It is mixed into counterfeit pills smuggled into the United States by the tens of millions. It is laced into many other drugs, such as meth, marijuana, and cocaine.[9] . . . The supplies of fentanyl and methamphetamine here have surpassed anything previously imaginable. These drugs come largely through a single source—Mexican traffickers—and, since 2019, have covered the United States."[10]

According to the US Drug Enforcement Agency (DEA), more than 95.5 million fentanyl-laced fake pills and nearly 12,000 pounds of fentanyl powder were seized by the agency in 2023. These seizures are the equivalent to more than 376.7 million lethal doses of fentanyl. A lethal dose is defined as 2 mg of fentanyl, which can kill a human of average weight. 2 mg is equal to just ten to fifteen grains of table salt.[11]

There are many communities across the United States in various stages of implementing elements of a Recovery Ready Community model. These communities are doing amazing work to stem the community impact of addiction. Many of these examples are cited in this book. There are also countless other communities in crisis trying to take the first steps to establish a cross-sector coalition and raise the prevention and recovery capital in their communities. This book specifically addresses the barriers to becoming a Recovery Ready Community and offers solutions to remove these barriers.

The book is intended for community leaders from all sectors, service providers, community-based organizations, academic institutions, individuals, and families. From this book, readers will understand the challenges facing communities across the United States in addressing the local impact of the epidemic of drug abuse, including public safety, public health, the local economy, and the social fabric that makes up the identity of the community.

Addiction and its impact is a community problem, and therefore needs to be addressed at the community level. While the federal and state governments enact policy and issue grants, it is up to the community to adopt these policies and secure these funds to confront addiction locally.

Again, this book is about hope. There *are* solutions to address addiction at the community level. This book provides a systematic and practical guide to becoming a Recovery Ready Community. It provides evidence-based information on the science of addiction and its roots in childhood trauma. Referencing examples such as the Greater Portsmouth Recovery Coalition (New Hampshire), Strafford County Addiction Task Force (New Hampshire), Lewiston-Auburn Area Recovery Collaborative (Maine), and other community coalitions, readers will learn how to build a community coalition, sustain the coalition over the long term, and deliver outcomes that benefit individuals, families, and communities alike.

Quinones, in his book *The Least of Us*, claims, "In a time when drug traffickers act like corporations and corporations act like traffickers, our best defense, perhaps our only defense, lies in bolstering community. America is strongest when we understand that we cannot succeed alone, and weakest when it's every man for himself."[12]

That same principle can be applied at the local community level. Instead of providers and community-based organizations competing for grants and prestige, community coalitions are perhaps the one place where collaborative spirit lives.

I have had the privilege of working alongside some of the most knowledgeable, compassionate, and intensely dedicated professionals and volunteers in my line of work. I have come to know dozens of thought leaders and authors with a lots of letters after their names signifying their education and certifications. However, sometimes the most insightful nugget of information comes from the person sitting across the table at a 12-step meeting, or the person in the passenger seat who asked for a ride, or the family in distress wondering how to convince their child to get help. The point is there are evidence-based best practices and there are real-life encounters. Both have a place at the table when discussing how to help people in need. Their stories are included in this book.

This book is organized into four sections, not including the appendix. Section 1 introduces the science of addiction, its roots in trauma, and the impact on individuals, families, and communities. Section 2 provides a roadmap to a solution to address the impact of addiction and trauma. Section 3 is a deep dive on the elements of a recovery ready community. And Section 4 provides a detailed case study on the Greater Portsmouth Recovery Coalition, a five-year coalition that continues to address the services, gaps, and barriers for individuals, families, and businesses in that community.

It is important to note that the guidance provided in this book is certainly not the only path to a Recovery Ready Community. However, the direction here is based on the collective lessons learned from several community coalitions.

Throughout the entirety of this book I speak as a person with lived experience, both as a person in long-term recovery from drug addiction and alcoholism, and as a professional in the recovery field. When I was discharged from Portsmouth Regional Hospital in 2012 following my admittance to the Behavioral Health Unit, there was no local support system. I had to board a plane to find treatment and recovery. Today that would not be the case. Portsmouth and the greater Seacoast region of New Hampshire stand as a shining example of a Recovery Ready Community.

—Mark Lefebvre, November, 2024

PROLOGUE

Mr. Hyde, from the Robert Louis Stevenson novella *The Strange Case of Dr. Jekyll and Mr. Hyde*, has been used as a metaphor for the struggles of addiction. Specifically, a person dealing with addiction often leads a double life—on one hand a father, husband, son, and brother of upstanding reputation, while on the other living a life of secrecy, dishonesty, and risky behavior. The individual will protect his addiction at all costs as the addiction can be a survival mechanism against untreated mental illness and childhood trauma.

But there is another side of Mr. Hyde that is less known. Mr. Hyde is human. He is real. And he is inherently aware of his struggles. He knows he leads a despicable life, and he hates himself for it. He is full of self-loathing. He is ashamed. He is scared. And there are days when death is the preferable alternative to suffering through another day as an active addict.

Mr. Hyde thrives on secrecy, lies, manipulation, and selfish behavior. He lives in the shadows. He was conceived by the marriage of untreated childhood trauma and opportunity. Like a messiah, Mr. Hyde was born to serve a higher purpose. He was born to fill the void—a void that resulted from being ill-equipped to deal with discomfort. He lacked the blueprint, the toolbox, or the manual for identifying and regulating his emotions. Mr. Hyde had the answers. Mr. Hyde had the goods. Mr. Hyde, in many ways, saved my life.

Conversely, what feeds Mr. Hyde can be taken away and replaced by transparency, honesty, and selflessness. His power is attenuated through love, humility, and service. The battle between starving and feeding Mr. Hyde is the fundamental conflict of the addict. This conflict is the choice addicts face every day between feeding or starving Mr. Hyde. The choice between a love affair with the addiction or with our recovery.

The individual who is in active addiction is not a bad person. He is a sick person who desperately wants to get better. It has been my experience that to understand oneself, to love oneself once again, the recovering addict must address the root causes that led him to seek the false promise of addiction. This is where the real work begins.

To the uninitiated, addiction is Hell without the companionship of Satan. The addict has no friends or loved ones when in the throes of active using. There are only marks to be conned, to be manipulated, to be used, to be milked dry, to serve. The pain evokes no words. The anguish leads to no sounds. The self-loathing falls on no ears.

Active addiction is a death sentence without the trial. There is no jury to judge. No lawyer to gently offer counsel. No counsel to counter the concept of the new reality. Or the revelation that without some miraculous intervention, there is no hope.

Addiction can also be a seductive temptress. Addiction can promise freedom from the unseen pain of untreated mental illness or trauma. In an ironic way, addiction can be useful as a coping mechanism. With that in mind, who are we to judge the motives of the active addict without knowing what is underneath the surface?

Addiction is not a choice. It is not a moral failing. The active addict needs his fix like the drowning swimmer needs a lifeline. It becomes a matter of survival—survival against the physical and mental torments of withdrawal. Fighting the craving is as futile as treading water with no hands or feet. There is no rescue without intervention.

There is a saying that knowledge is power. But with knowledge comes responsibility. Yes, addiction is a disease. Yes, we are sick people looking to get well. But are we *really* doing our part to get well? Are we working our recovery program to the best of our abilities? Are we making everyday decisions that set us up for success? And protecting the people we love?

We may not be able to control our future. However, the steps we take, the decisions we make at this moment, will lay the groundwork for our future. Every journey begins with the first step. Whether we have one day, one week, one month, or one year of recovery under our belts, each of us has taken that first lonely yet courageous step. Where that journey takes us is up to each of us.

Know that the end of your story has not yet been written.

SECTION 1

THE CHALLENGE

CHAPTER 1

UNDERSTANDING ADDICTION

Aaron was fidgety. As he sat in the front seat of my car, he expressed his gratitude for the ride to the Heroin Anonymous (HA) meeting at the Triangle Club in Dover. I noted to myself that he was not making eye contact with me as we engaged in small talk about the day. I asked if he planned to get his 30-day chip at the meeting, which incidentally was the first HA meeting in the state of New Hampshire.

Aaron had asked me to be his sponsor a few weeks prior. I was attending the HA meetings at the Triangle Club on a regular basis, giving rides to some of the young men who had no transportation. Aaron, a twenty-two-year-old from Seabrook, a husband and father, was one of these young men.

Modeled as an extension of the 12-step program of Alcoholics Anonymous, the Tuesday night HA meeting was a popular gathering of recovering heroin addicts from the Seacoast and Strafford County. Folks from neighboring Maine towns like Sanford, Lebanon, and Alfred would also attend. On any given Tuesday there could be as many as seventy attendees. The meeting offered chips for continuous lengths of sobriety—eleven months, ten months, counting down to thirty days and the "most important person in the room, not to single you out, but to welcome you in" 24-hour chip. The recognition of lengths of sobriety is important not only to the recipient, but also for others in the room to show that the program works.

At the meeting Aaron shuffled to the podium when the 30-day chip roll call was called by the meeting "chip person." Amid the applause and words of encouragement, Aaron returned to his seat without looking up. My spidey senses were aroused.

On the way back to Seabrook, Aaron shared that he had had a relapse a day earlier but was too ashamed to talk about it before the meeting. A floodlight triggered on as we pulled into his driveway. We sat in silence for a few minutes before I could muster what I thought were the right words of encouragement that tomorrow would be another day. As he got out of the car, I shook his hand, gave him a pat on the back and asked him to check in with me in the morning.

On the way home I stopped at a CVS and bought Aaron a card to again offer words of encouragement. I scribbled the following message on the card: *Aaron, a quick note to say*

I've been thinking of you. Remember, it is not how many times we fall that defines us. Rather, it is how many times we get up. Call me when you're ready. —Mark

I never had the opportunity to give Aaron the card. Aaron, twenty-two years of age, husband, father, son, outdoorsman, and student, died of a heroin overdose on Tuesday, October 13, 2015 at his home. I still have that card in my office.

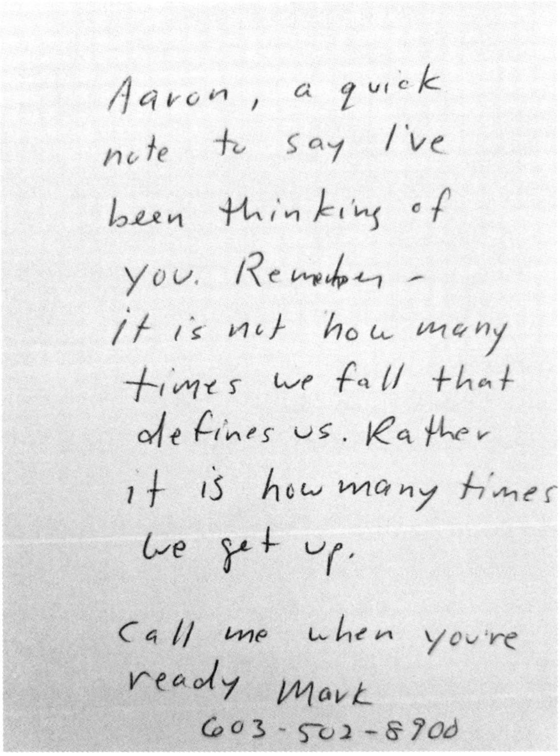

Figure 1: My note to Aaron, days before his fatal overdose.

Addiction in the United States

According to the US Surgeon General's Report on Alcohol, Drugs, and Health, "the vast majority of people in the United States who misuse substances do not have substance use disorders."[13] Regardless, substance use can put individual users and others around them at risk of harm, whether or not they have a disorder. "Also, early initiation, substance use, and substance use disorders are associated with a variety of negative consequences, including deteriorating relationships, poor school performance, loss of employment, diminished mental health, and increases in sickness and death (e.g., motor vehicle crashes, poisoning, violence, or accidents). It is therefore critical to prevent the full spectrum of substance use problems in addition to treating those with substance use disorders."[14]

As we will see later in this section, in addition to the tragic loss of life across the country, addiction affects individuals, families, and communities in different ways. Lives are lost, families are shattered, and communities face threats to economic vitality, public health, and public safety.

Addiction 101

As a child growing up in the 1960s and 1970s, societal norms informed me that addiction was bad and scary, a modern-day scarlet A. Musicians such as Jimi Hendrix, Janis Joplin, and Gram Parsons each succumbed to their dependence on substances in their musical prime, which reinforced the message that drugs were bad, and they were deadly if taken in excess.

Exploitation films including *Reefer Madness* (1936) and *The Pace That Kills* (1935) sensationalized the subculture of drug use in pre- and post-war America with campy if not outrageous depictions of people who chose to use drugs. Like many others from my generation, I grew up with a great sense of fear of drugs. For me, this fear inevitably evolved to fascination, which led to curiosity, which led to recreational drug use, which led to addiction. Despite these media-informed childhood influences, I never succumbed to the common misconceptions that people who used drugs were deviants. Nor did I believe drug users were criminals who should be punished.

The National Institute on Drug Abuse (NIDA) defines addiction as "a chronic, relapsing disorder characterized by compulsive drug seeking and use despite adverse consequences. It (addiction) is considered a brain disorder because it involves functional changes to brain circuits involved in reward, stress, and self-control. Those changes may last a long time after a person has stopped taking drugs."[15]

The American Society of Addiction Medicine (ASAM) defines addiction as "a treatable, chronic medical disease involving complex interactions among brain circuits, genetics, the environment, and an individual's life experiences. People with addiction use substances or engage in behaviors that become compulsive and often continue despite harmful consequences."[16]

Under the fifth edition of the American Psychiatric Association's Diagnostic and Statistical Manual (DSM-5), substance use disorders (SUD) can be diagnosed when individuals meet at least two of eleven criteria (symptoms), each of which falls into one of four categories[17]:

1. Impaired social control
2. Social problems

3. Risky use

4. Physical dependence

Based on the number of diagnostic criteria met, SUDs are categorized as mild (2-3), moderate (4-5), or severe (6 or more). Experts generally concur that severe SUD most closely aligns with what is commonly thought of as addiction. Through screening, mild to moderate SUD can be identified and addressed before it becomes severe. The eleven criteria are:

1. Using in larger amounts or for longer than intended

2. Wanting to cut down/stop using, but not managing to

3. Spending a lot of time to get/use/recover from use

4. Craving

5. Inability to manage commitments due to use

6. Continuing to use, even when it causes problems in relationships

7. Giving up important activities because of use

8. Continuing to use, even when it puts you in danger

9. Continuing to use, even when physical or psychological problems may be made worse by use

10. Increasing tolerance

11. Withdrawal symptoms

Why do people use drugs? Some use drugs for the effect, as drugs can produce intense feelings of pleasure. People who use drugs often chase the feeling of that first euphoric high from their first use of a given drug. Many people use drugs recreationally without that use leading to addiction. I am not one of them.

Under proper medical care, drugs help us cope with a number of mental illnesses including anxiety, depression, and trauma. For others, drugs enhance physical or mental performance and allow us to better focus. Performance-enhancing drugs (PEDs), and amphetamines are examples. Others, especially adolescents and young adults, use drugs because of peer pressure and a desire to fit in.[18]

In her book *The Recovering*, Leslie Jamison encapsulates the essence of why we pick up. "It's nothing new, the desire to disrupt consciousness—to soften it, blunt it, sharpen it, distort, flood it with bliss, paper over its disenchantments. It's a way to describe the act of living. We just keep discovering things we can put into our bodies to change ourselves more dramatically, more suddenly: to feel relief or euphoria or the dulling of anxiety, to feel *different*. . ."[19]

The obvious question is why do we need to feel this way? What secrets are we protecting? What pain are we trying to numb, what hole are we trying to fill, what trauma are we trying to escape from? Before we correlate the impact of many of the root causes of substance use, including untreated mental illness, we need to understand the science of addiction.

Addiction and the Brain

In a podcast interview with master licensed addiction counselor (MLADC) John Iudice, he and I discussed the changes that occur in the brain during active addiction.

"I think a good way to explain how our natural reward system works is that it is a process that is universally human. Everyone has dopamine, oxytocin, and some of the other neurotransmitters that are more commonly associated with substance use. People who use drugs develop a different relationship with the experiences that give them those neurotransmitters," said Iudice. "Dopamine is what makes you get up and go eat a meal, it's the motivation required to do anything. Most of us can relate to having a craving or an urge to go get something that we enjoy. What's happening is that the neurotransmitter dopamine is being released in the brain and in the body." [20]

Iudice continued, "Oxytocin is the other neurotransmitter that is commonly released with opiate use. I've heard countless people explain it as the same feeling as getting a hug, or specifically, that comfort, that warm, safe feeling that comes from being nurtured, or being hugged by someone you really care about. That's a common experience that isn't quite as extreme as taking an opiate, as you're not going to get the rush the same way. But all humans experience that natural release of oxytocin from our human experience."[21]

"I Thought I Would Die"

When in the throes of my opioid addiction I chased the feeling of the first high I experienced with prescribed pain medication, long before anyone had heard of oxycontin. I was administered Vicodin (hydrocodone) following knee surgery in my early twenties and felt a euphoria that I can only explain as an abstract collage of warmth, safety, confidence, and surrender. And intense joy. Unspeakable joy.

Dr. Alex Elswick, a researcher at the University of Kentucky, explains his own experience with opioids. "When I did opioids at eighteen, I experienced a huge and unnatural dopaminergic response. The more evolved part of my brain knew the consequences of using, but that didn't matter to my limbic system. All it cared about is survival, which meant all it cared about is how much dopamine it's receiving. The sensation was so strong that nothing else mattered. That's why people who are addicted to opiates forego food, water, bonding, sex, and everything else. So, if you think talking about right and wrong and better choices will make a difference, think again."[22]

Over the course of my adulthood, I've had a number of surgeries that required pain medication, in some cases for a week or more following surgery. Some of these surgeries required intensive pain treatment including Percocet (oxycodone), morphine, Demerol (meperidine), and eventually OxyContin. To put a finer point on Dr. Elswick's comment about making better choices, during my active addiction I would actually look forward to the surgery in anticipation of eventually being prescribed pain medication. And when the prescriptions expired, or when my doctor refused to prescribe a refill, I would inevitably experience the misery of withdrawal. At that time, I was incapable of making better choices. I thought I would die.

Tolerance and Withdrawal

As a person who uses drugs increases the amount of their drug of choice or the frequency of use, their tolerance to the drug can be affected. Again, John Iudice offers a clinical explanation: "What happens during withdrawal is that when a person doesn't get as much of that neurotransmitter, the body's natural attempt at correcting it is to temper the release of those neurotransmitters. And what ends up happening is someone will take more, and they are not getting the same effect. They don't get the warm hug feeling from maybe taking 10 milligrams of something. So now they'll take 30 milligrams, or they'll try to ingest it in other ways that will make the experience more intense again, just so they can get back to that point of having that 'normal' effect. That's a slippery slope because eventually they get to a point where their body is going to react to the consumption of that additional dosage. That's a sign that they are getting closer to that place where they experience more severe addiction and physiological dependence is starting to happen through tolerance and withdrawal."[23]

I've heard many in recovery say that their fear of withdrawal is far greater than their desire to use. I know this is certainly my own experience and perspective. Iudice explains why. "When someone is in the throes of active addiction, withdrawal can be one of most horrific experiences because of the intense level of physical pain and emotional restlessness that someone who uses drugs is experiencing. It's the body's adjustment to having had a certain level of exposure to the substance that person has been ingesting from outside sources. The body gets sick without having that substance. That person needs that external substance in order to make themselves feel better again. And it's hard to get through."

From the user's perspective, withdrawal, and eliminating the symptoms of withdrawal, can almost feel as though their experience is a matter of life and death. Legitimate fear of real survival. This helps us better understand and hopefully empathize with the decisions facing a person in that survival state. Is repeated drug usage a choice? Or is it behavior that prolongs survival? This notion of choice and behavior in turn helps us to understand some of the controversial elements of the recovery continuum such as stigma, harm reduction, and medication-assisted treatment.

Back to my conversation with Iudice. John posed the following scenario and rhetorical question: "If I feel as though I'm not going to survive this withdrawal, it's a matter of survival for me to get that next drug. I'm only putting that out there. Not so much to be difficult for you and me as people in recovery to talk about, but for other folks that are either family members or loved ones, or affected others, to kind of understand at a very layman's level what may be going on with that individual that you care about. They feel as though in order for them to survive, they need to get to that place where they can take that pain away. It is a really important reminder that they're not trying to hurt themselves, or even when they seem upset, they're not choosing to be going through that experience. They've gotten to a point where the choice has been more and more removed from the equation over time.

"So armed with that knowledge, what can the rest of us do in addition to being aware of that dynamic, but to be supportive, or to get that person help in a way that is compassionate toward those that we care for that may be going through that situation?"

Cravings and Obsession

As a recovering addict and alcoholic, I can speak firsthand about the phenomenon of craving. From the first sip of an alcoholic beverage or the first hit off a joint, I would be thinking of the next. I would want more before I'd had any.

The DSM-5 considers craving to be the driving force behind the compulsion to use drugs. Craving brings forth the "memory of a pleasant experience superimposed on a negative emotional state such as depression, anxiety, trauma, or other similar mental state," and is the motivational drive in addiction.[24]

Brittany Reichmann, statewide business advisor for Maine's Recovery Friendly Workplace program, and who is a person in long-term recovery from an SUD, offers her perspective: "It is a difficult thing to explain the phenomenon of craving to individuals who have not experienced substance use disorder. I would chase and chase that next high, regardless of the consequences. My intentions never aligned with my actions. I never wanted to hurt anyone, yet repeatedly I would engage in behaviors that hurt the people who loved me. Whether that was stealing or lying, no price was too high to pay. It is a very irrational process, even though we now know scientifically it makes sense. It may never make sense to the people looking in from the outside."[25]

For people who use drugs, that first high can be so powerful that we seek that first sensational experience each time we use. Hence the obsessive behavior. That feeling, however, is often elusive for a number of physiological reasons. That chase is the reason most of us cannot stop despite the negative consequences. The cravings lead to obsessive behaviors and rituals surrounding our addiction. *How many pills do I have left? Where am I going to score my next fix? How am I going to pay for it?*

Addiction Rooted in Childhood Trauma

Gabor Maté, noted author on the subject of addiction, states that "not all addictions are rooted in abuse or trauma, but I do believe they can all be traced to painful experience. A hurt is at the center of *all* addictive behaviors."[26]

For me, my addictive behavior was largely due to untreated childhood trauma. I wrote the following passage at the age of sixty-five shortly after experiencing a transient ischemic attack (TIA), also sometimes known as a "mini stroke." Shortly after the TIA, I began to experience dissociative episodes, which in turn led to vivid images of experiences from my childhood. At that time, I had been sober for over twelve years. My therapist asked me to write an essay that described these experiences. I include this essay to qualify as a trauma survivor.

Time Travel in Silent Sadness

A parallel universe exists in my unconscious mind within which my repressed thoughts and memories beckon me. When I visit this space, I have the ability to visualize patterns, light, colors, and shapes that trigger a kaleidoscope of recall from my lockbox of traumatic experiences, dangerous thoughts, and deepest dreams. These visions evoke my deepest and clearest visceral emotions in a manner that defies explanation. While in deep meditation, the best I can do to explain this phenomenon is to attach the emotion of sadness; however, that one-dimensional seven-letter word is nothing more than a mere label, a tag, a temporary clue that enables me to preserve that momentary experience as a permanent record deep in my unconsciousness. All said, the wave of that ill-described sense of melancholy is overwhelming for me.

Some of these places I envision seem so real that I'm fooled into thinking that I've actually been there before. Perhaps I have been there in a metaphysical sense, whatever that might be. I see blankets of clouds with shapes and shades of gray and white that defy description. In my mind I've seen these clouds before at this precise time of day in a familiar place that is far, far away. There is no other way to explain it. I see sunny skies that spray shadows on the landscape surrounding me that bring me to familiar places that, ironically, I've never visited in this world. But to me, they are as real as the view outside my window. These recollections are often triggered by a state of deep meditation.

The melancholy is comforting to me for reasons I cannot yet explain. In his landmark book, The Body Keeps the Score, *Dr. Bessel van der Kolk posits that "trauma affects the entire human-organism—body, mind, and brain. In PTSD, the body continues to defend against a threat that belongs to the past."[27] Does the sadness I feel when experiencing these visions stem from some unresolved trauma? And does the comfort I feel from the sadness stem from some unexplained method of self-preservation? These questions remain unanswered to this day.*

What happened?

At the age of fourteen I witnessed the gruesome death of a friend. As a child I went into shock and have no recollection of the immediate aftermath, nor the twelve or so hours that transpired afterwards. At that time, I never resolved the shock or grief stemming from that event with my parents, teachers, or any healthcare provider. The next morning after learning that my friend succumbed from these injuries, my parents sent me to school that day. I sobbed uncontrollably at the bus stop while my schoolmates tried to console me.

At the age of eighteen while away for my freshman year in college, I was told that my younger brother had cancer. A year later, he went into remission. Two years later, we learned that the cancer had returned and that it was incurable. Five months later, my brother succumbed to cancer at the age of eighteen with me at his side. Once again, at that time I never resolved my grief over the loss of my brother with my parents or any healthcare provider. The day following his burial I returned to school. My studies and my fledgling addictions were my coping mechanisms.

Perhaps the comfort I feel in sadness is that it is MY sadness. It is an unfortunate part of my identity, a defense mechanism to mask the residual pain from my traumatic past that is still not completely resolved. I feel the secrets of my past lie somewhere deep in those places within my unconscious mind.

I stopped using drugs and alcohol over twelve years ago. For a time, drugs afforded me respite from my pain. However, they failed to resolve the *source* of that pain. Has sadness replaced my addictions? Or is sadness a byproduct of my unconscious journeys, and therefore a productive step of stripping away the façade, or what I call the "lockbox" I've built to store these traumatic events?

I've told my therapist that these journeys feel like I'm tripping. I am detached from, but simultaneously drawn to the visions like a moth to flame. The journeys leave me exhausted and at times, feeling confused. I obsess over them for days.

Dr. van der Kolk suggests that we "dare to tell the truth" about our traumatic experiences. Through years of therapy I've learned that talking about these feelings and the triggers that activate them can help take away their power. I've learned that we are only as sick as our secrets.

As a master trainer for ACE Interface, I now know the correlations between high ACEs (adverse childhood experiences) scores and substance use disorder. As someone with a high ACE score, I now understand that as a population, people with an ACEs score of 4 or more (out of 10), are:

- 12 times more at risk for suicide

- 7 times more likely to develop alcoholism

- 4 times more likely to develop depression

- 2–4 times higher risk of using alcohol or other drugs

- 2–4 times more likely to begin substance use at a young age

- 2 times higher rate of heart disease or lung cancer[28]

German-born teacher and spiritual leader Eckhart Tolle writes, "One of the main tasks of the mind is to fight or remove that emotional pain, which is one of the reasons for its incessant activity, but all it can ever achieve is to cover it up temporarily. In fact, the harder the mind struggles to get rid of the pain, the greater the pain. The mind can never find the solution, nor can it afford to allow you to find the solution, because it is itself an intrinsic part of the 'problem.'"[29]

Gabor Maté concurs. "At the core of every addiction is an emptiness based in abject fear. The addict dreads and abhors the present moment; she bends feverishly only toward the next time, the moment when her brain, infused with her drug of choice, will briefly experience itself as liberated from the burden of the past and the fear of the future—the two elements that make the present intolerable."[30]

Co-Occurring Mental Illness

The simultaneous presence of both a mental illness and a substance use disorder is known as a co-occurring disorder and is common among people in treatment for substance use disorder. According to SAMHSA, co-occurring disorders may include any combination of two or more substance use disorders, and mental disorders identified in the DSM-5.[31]

People with mental illness are more likely to experience a substance use disorder than those not affected by a mental illness. According to SAMHSA's 2022 National Survey on Drug Use and Health, approximately 21.5 million adults in the United States have a co-occurring disorder. More than one in four adults living with serious mental health problems also have a co-occurring SUD. Substance use problems occur more frequently with certain mental health problems, including depression, anxiety disorders, schizophrenia, or personality disorders.[32]

For individuals with co-occurring disorders, it is vital that treatment considers both the mental illness and substance use disorder holistically, especially if either or both are being treated with medications. According to John Iudice, "It can be really important to have mental health therapy combined with the use of medication as it helps the individual adjust to the initial phases of taking medication. It also helps someone stay on routine with taking the medications at the right time and as prescribed."[33]

Diane Fontneau, MS, LCMHC and MLADC, is the clinical director at Dismas Home, a women's transitional recovery home in Manchester, New Hampshire. When interviewed for the podcast series *It Takes a Village: Addiction Prevention & Recovery on the Seacoast*, Fontneau was a clinical manager at Seacoast Mental Health Center. "I think that we used to look at things in silos whereby it was mental health, or it was substance use, and people with clinical master's degrees either treated mental health or substance use, and never the two shall meet. The truth is that they did meet, and people were seeing two different providers for a condition that, with proper training, could be treated at the same time."[34]

When asked what providers are doing differently today for co-occurring patients, Fontneau replied, "I think Seacoast Mental Health Center does a good job of treating people with co-occurring disorders in having well-trained practitioners and prescribers who do research and weigh out the benefits, pros, and cons of medications they're prescribing, and how are they going to interact. They monitor what people are using, and make sure people are safe. SMHC is not a punitive program for substance use disorders; we really use a harm reduction approach in that we're not going to kick anyone out for testing positive for a substance. We're going to work on both mental health and SUD symptoms simultaneously to provide the best help."

Addiction and the Family

Nancy (not her real name) is forty-three years old, and the mother of a two-year-old daughter. Nancy grew up about twenty-five miles north of Boston. When Nancy was eleven, her mother died at the age of thirty-eight from liver failure that was medically attributed to years of alcohol abuse. Her mother left Nancy and her eight-year-old brother Anthony behind.

Nancy recalls, "I saw some stuff; I experienced some stuff at a very young age that no person should experience. I don't think I understood then that she was an alcoholic, so I didn't understand that aspect of her being a drunk or not fully with faculties. But I do remember we went to the liquor store regularly, and that she would buy two big jugs of wine to last the week, usually two of the gallon-size bottles of red wine. I was probably ten at the time, but I remember."

Nancy recalls that she'd find her mother passed out on the floor during the day after her mom missed picking her and her brother up from school. There were other times when she could not wake her mom, and Nancy would prepare dinner for her and her brother while their father was still at work.

"She ended up having liver failure and liver problems that made her stomach really distended. And I can remember one day sitting with her, and I asked her, 'Mom, are you pregnant?' Because her belly was big and round."

Nancy's mom replied, "No."

"Are you dying?"

Nancy's mom said, "Yes. And she made like a sad face, and I was like, okay, and that was that."

"I'm eleven years old and my mom just told me she's dying."

Nancy still lives with that trauma today, more than thirty years later. Her brother Anthony refuses to discuss it. [35]

Actual 911 call[36]

Lest there be no doubt that addiction is a family disease, consider an abbreviated version of an exchange between a mother, her friend, and a 911 dispatcher from Madison County in central Kentucky.

Dispatcher: "911, what's your emergency?"

Nikki: "I need someone at my apartment. My son has overdosed."

. . .

Friend: "He's overdosed. I think he may be gone."

Nikki Strunck's son Brendan Strunck died in January, 2016 at age twenty-four, succumbing to his drug addiction that began when he was thirteen years old.

For every individual having a substance use disorder, several others including family members, friends, and fellow workers are also impacted. According to the report *The Ripple Effect: The Impact of the Opioid Epidemic on Children and Families*, an individual's substance use disorder sends ripples through families and communities, and ignoring these ripples can cause long-lasting consequences.[37]

Based on that report's studies, there are eight million children in the United States living in a household with at least one parent with a substance use disorder. The impact can include disrupted lives, problems in schools, trauma, and the potential accidental use of drugs in the home by children and family pets.

Kinship caregivers, or angels as they are often called, warrant a deeper recognition as family members who have stepped in to care for their grandchildren, siblings, nieces, and nephews. Denyse Richter of Portsmouth, New Hampshire, founded Step Up Parents, a nonprofit agency that provides direct financial support to families in New Hampshire and southern Maine. She explains, "We help families who are providing kinship care for children who have parents with a substance use disorder. These children have been placed in kinship care with a member of their family, be they an aunt, uncle, grandparent, and sometimes even friends of family who are considered to be family members. And it's unfortunate that the parents of these children may be incarcerated or in treatment, or unfortunately in some cases, they are deceased. Every request we receive is different, and every family is different. But all have a similar underlying substance use disorder within the family that is making life hard for the family, and specifically for the children we're trying to help."[38]

"A Tornado Has Gone Through My Life"

I shared previously that I was admitted to the Portsmouth Behavioral Unit at Portsmouth (New Hampshire) Regional Hospital in 2012. My not-so-secret life of addiction and alcohol abuse was finally exposed to my family, our relatives, my employer, and our close friends. I was admitted to the unit out of concern that I would harm myself over the guilt and shame I felt for my actions.

My wife Vivian shared what this experience was like for her during a recent podcast that we recorded together: "I remember a story from Al-Anon where it talked about a farmer and his wife who were hiding in the basement of their farm because a tornado was striking the farm. When the storm was over, they came upstairs, and they looked around and the farm was in complete shambles. Everything was gone, everything was broken, everything was dead, it was just a mess. And the farmer said to his wife, well, good news is, the storm is over. But the reality is, the work is only just beginning. The carnage is still there. And that's kind of how I felt. When you had gone to the hospital. It's like, okay, the storm is over. But a tornado has gone through my life. So that (treatment) was just the beginning."[39]

During that period of the early 2010s, there were very few resources for individuals like me to find local or even regional treatment following release from initial detoxification. And there were even fewer resources for families to get the support they need for their recovery. One of the very few resources was the New Hampshire chapter of NAMI (National Alliance on Mental Illness), which provided local education and networking. Vivian used this resource to learn more about addiction as a family disease.

Vivian and I were very resourceful in 2012. We researched extensively for resources to help us recover individually and as a couple. Fast-forward to today and there is a wide and varied network of professional services, community-based organizations, and peer groups to support families in New Hampshire, and across the United States.

GRASP (Grief Recovery After Substance Passing)

Grief affects each of us in different ways. For every individual who loses their life from addiction, just like with any disease, we experience different emotions at different phases of our grief over time. There is obviously *sadness* that stems from loss. Sadness can intensify as the reality of loss sinks in. There is *anger* that can be directed at the person who passed, family members, healthcare professionals, and even God. *Guilt* naturally surfaces as survivors wonder if they could have done more to prevent the death of a loved one. *Fear* is another common emotion that stems from uncertainty about the future. Finally, *loneliness* is perhaps the most enduring of the grief emotions. The sense of being alone, especially during holidays and anniversaries, or even everyday situations that were perhaps shared with that loved one.

New Hampshire is fortunate to have several chapters of the nationwide support group, GRASP (Grief Recovery After Substance Passing) which was founded to offer peer support among grieving family members of individuals who have passed due to substance use. The program offers understanding, compassion, and support to help surviving family members deal with the grief, guilt, and even shame that often accompanies substance use in the family. From their website: "Grief Recovery After Substance Passing (GRASP) was created to offer understanding, compassion, and support for those who have lost someone they love through addiction and overdose . . . We walk it together; hand in hand and heart to heart."[40]

Heather Blumenfeld leads the Seacoast (New Hampshire) GRASP chapter and chairs bimonthly meetings at the Triangle Club in Dover. These meetings are open only to families who have lost a loved one to addiction. "Grief is a process you have to go through. So many people push grief down and do not allow themselves to begin the process. Being in a safe place with other people going through a similar passing encourages people to start that process and begin to heal," she said. "I went through it too. I used to dread these meetings. It's hard to get yourself to that meeting, but you feel so much lighter when you leave. You really do. You're leaving your baggage to the power of the group, even if you sit and cry for half of the meeting, you feel better when you leave."[41]

Stigmatizing Drug Users and their Families

In her book *The Recovering*, author Leslie Jamison explains, "every addiction story wants a villain. But America has never been able to decide whether the addicts are victims or criminals, whether addiction is an illness or a crime."[42] Compounding the false narrative of drug use in America is the impact of the so-called War on Drugs, a campaign that was both covert (Harry Anslinger) and overt (Reagan administration). Anslinger established the notorious Narcotics Farm in Lexington, Kentucky in 1935, which was the very first drug treatment center in the United States. The farm housed the famous—author William S. Burroughs and musicians Chet Baker and Sonny Rollins—but more often than not, the forgotten and marginalized. It is important to note that Anslinger led the national fearmongering about drugs and drug users, which in turn led to the development of US policy that considered drug users criminals and deviants. This narrative and the ensuing US policies were mainly intended to marginalize people of color, and it continued through the end of the twentieth century.

The Reagan administration, and specifically Nancy Reagan, famously launched the Just Say No campaign in 1983,[43] which often involved local law enforcement visiting elementary and grade schools to convey the message that encouraged kids to "just say no" if offered drugs. These well-meaning officers typically referred to drug users and dealers as losers and bums, which served as a warning to children that they too risk becoming a loser or a bum.

The impact on communities resulting from the War on Drugs has been devastating, especially in the middle of the national opioid epidemic. According to Dr. Brendan Saloner in his paper *Public Health Strategy for the Opioid Crisis*, the national dialog around opioids has been dominated by several approaches that on their own are inadequate or harmful. From their paper, Saloner et al. highlight the negative impact to communities stemming from the War on Drugs including "long-term scarring effects on communities," creating the misconception "that drug use is a moral failing," and "fail[ing] to recognize the role of trauma and adverse childhood experiences in addiction."[44]

Dr. Brandon del Pozo, a former New York City police officer and former chief of police in Burlington, Vermont, has conducted research on the government's response to addiction. Del Pozo states, "The war on drugs has been an enduring and monumental failure, afflicting Black and brown Americans out of all proportion, not to mention drawing the nation's police officers into an endless cycle of futility and burnout. Drugs are as accessible as ever and have only gotten more potent—increasing people's risk of overdose and making it harder for them to recover and lead stable, productive lives."[45]

Stigma and discriminating language affects not only the individual, but the family as well, often preventing anyone from seeking help. We will address methods to overcome the stigma though community outreach and education in Chapter 13.

Addiction and the Community

In New Hampshire, the state medical examiner issues a monthly report that tracks monthly and yearly trends for Narcan, opioid-related emergency department (ED) visits, emergency management specialists (EMS) calls, treatment admissions, and overdose deaths. As of August 16, 2024, overdose deaths for the period of January 1, 2024 through July 31, 2024 in New Hampshire have declined over 10 percent (170 vs. 198). Likewise, EMS incidents and Narcan administrations, are also down significantly compared to the same period in 2023.[46]

Author Sam Quinones, in his wonderfully provocative *The Least of Us*, the follow-up book to *Dreamland*, his groundbreaking expose of the Mexican cartels and big pharma, offers his view on the impact of addiction on the community. "We used to believe people needed to hit rock bottom before seeking treatment. That's another idea made obsolete by our addiction crisis and the current synthetic drug supply. It belongs to an era when drugs were merciful. Nowadays, people are living in tents, screaming at unseen demons, raped, pimped, beaten, unshowered, and unfed. That would seem to be rock bottom. Yet it's not enough to persuade people to get treatment."[47]

Substance use in the United States has had a devastating impact to the community, affecting public health (transmission of infectious diseases, discarded needles), public safety (crime, housing insecurity), and the local economy (absenteeism, disability). The opioid crisis in particular has put pressure on the healthcare system with overdoses, overdose reversals through naloxone administration, increased emergency room visits and EMS calls. In terms of total impact on communities, such statistics only tell part of the story.

The Economic Impact of Addiction

The economic impact of the nation's opioid crisis is staggering. In addition to the toll on families and loved ones, opioid use imposes significant costs for communities across the country. The Joint Economic Committee of the US Senate estimates the opioid epidemic cost $1.04 trillion in 2018, $985 billion in 2019 and nearly $1.5 trillion in 2020. The rise in fatal opioid overdoses in 2021 and 2022 suggests the total cost likely increased during that period.[48]

The impact of substance use disorders in the workplace is profound. In July 2023, *Fortune* magazine reported that over forty-six million American workers struggle with substance use disorder and issued a warning to businesses to act.[49] According to the Federal Recovery-Ready Workplace Interagency Workgroup, nearly twenty-seven million Americans aged eighteen and older with a diagnosed substance use disorder were employed, of which 77.6 percent (20.9 million) worked full-time.[50]

In response to the staggering economic cost of addiction in the United States, the Biden-Harris Administration unveiled resources to equip businesses with tools to expand employment opportunities for the tens of millions of Americans seeking recovery from substance use disorders.[51] This national "Recovery-Ready Workplace" initiative is modeled after New Hampshire's pioneering Recovery Friendly Workplace program launched by Governor Sununu in 2018.

CHAPTER 2

ADVERSE CHILDHOOD EXPERIENCES

Is Dad Okay?

My neighborhood was sleepy this hot July afternoon, and the sticky air hung like a festoon of Spanish moss in a Mississippi bayou. The creak of crickets and the drone of cicada added to the made-up image in my mind of a Southern summer day. Just running from my friend's mother's car to the front stoop of our three-story tenement caused my loose-fitting t-shirt to stick to my skin. I had spent much of the morning and early afternoon swimming at my friend's house farther down the street and near the town line. His mom generously offered to give me a ride home, thus saving my parents the trip.

After waving goodbye to my friend from our front porch I opened the screen door and ran up the steps to the door to our second-floor apartment. My family occupied the top two floors of the building with my maternal grandparents, who owned the building, living on the ground level. Because their door was closed, I assumed that my grandparents were out for the afternoon. I also noticed that our door was closed and locked, which was also unusual if my parents were home. Perhaps they were out back in our own swimming pool.

Over a bowl of Cheerios earlier that morning I learned that my father had a rare Saturday off. Between his job as a firefighter and moonlighting as a short-haul truck driver, we typically would not see him until late afternoon on Saturdays. Oh well, he's earned it, I thought to myself.

Turning the doorknob to our apartment door, I found it locked. This was highly unusual, even if everyone was down at the pool out back. As I was about to descend the stairs to check the backyard, I heard the door open softly with my mother's hand holding the door close to her body. I turned and peered into the space in the door and noticed the entire apartment was dark. My curiosity must have been evident on my facial expression, so before I had a chance to speak, my mother put a finger to her pursed lips and said, "Shh . . . your father is not feeling well. Your uncle is here sitting with him."

My twelve-year-old mind raced, catastrophizing the situation. I mulled the facts in a microsecond of rational thought. Door locked. Lights off. Shades drawn. Uncle here. None of this made sense to me.

I looked up to my mother, who towered more than two feet above me in the space she allowed in the doorway. Her face was pressed against the door. "What's wrong with him?" I asked.

"He's having a bad migraine. Your uncle is sitting with him," she repeated.

This also made no sense to me. My father had had migraines in the past. We never pulled the shades down before, nor did this ever require a visit from my uncle. Concerned that something was really wrong, my mind started racing. Looking back into my mother's eyes for some, any signal of reassurance, I panicked.

"Is he going to die?" I asked earnestly, not really wanting to know.

What occurred next was so sudden, so unthinkable, that I was completely taken by surprise. Without uttering a word, my mother slapped me across the face with such force that it snapped my head sideways. I nearly fell down the stairs in the shock of that violent moment.

"Don't you ever say that again," she admonished, slamming the door shut.

I sat on the top step and felt the sting of the slap begin to fade, but that was not what pained me. I was baffled as to why my mother resorted to hitting me when all I was seeking was some reassurance that my father was going to be okay.

As a kid, I never asked my mother about this event. What was the point? Would she remember? Would she be remorseful? Or would she hit me again for bringing it up?

Looking back on this event decades later, I now know that a twelve-year-old boy learned that day that it was not safe to express himself in situations where he felt emotionally vulnerable. At that time I learned that keeping my thoughts to myself was a safer route. And that discomfort to express myself plagues me to this day.

The Impact of Childhood Trauma

I hit my children exactly once in their childhood. They were fighting about some sibling crisis across from each other's bedroom, upstairs from where I was working in the study. After numerous warnings to solve their issues peacefully, I lost my shit and bounded up the stairs to give each a whack with my hand on their behinds.

The look of terror on their faces in reaction froze me in my tracks. I had crossed a line I swore I would never cross. In that moment I saw my father's right arm swing high with a leather strap in hand. In that moment I felt the sting of my mother's hand on my cheek. In their eyes I saw the terror I felt while cowering, waiting for my turn to be whipped on the bare bottom. No child should fear their parents. I never want my kids to be afraid of me ever again.

Many of us in the field of recovery have learned about childhood trauma and the correlation between high ACEs scores and mental health and substance use later in life. Through the publication of the work of Drs. Vincent Felitti and Robert Anda from the early 1990s, we were introduced to three categories of adverse childhood experiences:

Household Dysfunction

1. Substance use

2. Parental separation or divorce

3. Mental illness in the family

4. Violence

5. Incarceration

Neglect

6. Emotional

7. Physical

Abuse

8. Emotional

9. Physical

10. Sexual

This study of more than seventeen thousand participants became known as the Adverse Childhood Experiences (ACEs) Study,[52] which demonstrated that childhood trauma is a primary case of "downstream" behavioral and health issues later in life. These issues include but are not limited to risky behaviors such as smoking, teenage pregnancy, alcoholism, substance use, and suicide. Health issues include heart disease, stroke, depression, and anxiety.

One of the key findings from the study is that toxic stress in the developmental years of early childhood has significant effects on the structure and function of the child's brain as he ages until his early twenties. ACEs are tallied for a score of 0-10. The Anda/Felitti study showed that individuals with an ACEs score of 4 or higher were twelve times more likely to have attempted suicide, seven times more likely to be alcoholic, and ten times more likely to have injected street drugs.[53]

In 2020, Pinetree Institute of Eliot, Maine and Portsmouth, New Hampshire, received funding from Rotary District 7780 to sponsor a three-year training program that provided master training of ACE Interface programming for nearly thirty volunteers. These community volunteers in turn were deployed to provide free ACEs training across Rockingham and Strafford counties in New Hampshire, and southern York County in Maine. The objective was to raise awareness and understanding of the impact of childhood trauma as a root cause of issues we were seeing in our homes, schools, and community.

Pinetree Institute invited Dr. Anda and Laura Porter, co-founders of the ACE Interface program, to conduct the master training. ACE Interface develops and disseminates educational products and empowerment strategies that help leaders throughout the nation to dramatically improve population health.

According to Dr. Larry McCullough, executive director of Pinetree Institute, and an ACE Interface master trainer himself, "ACEs has a huge impact on health issues later in life, and is connected to things you would expect, like mental health, but also things like substance use disorder, addiction, heart disease, smoking, financial stress, and even days missed from work. Therefore, if we start to understand childhood trauma and its impact, then we can start to address prevention with parents and with the children themselves in order to improve our quality of life as adults."[54]

Due to the dramatic advancements in scientific research of the brain made possible with imaging technology, scientists can now see how the brain develops.[55] We know that the human brain is a complex and ever-changing structure within the human body. Especially in childhood, the human brain can alter its structure to adapt to experiences.[56] Adverse childhood experiences have been shown to have a profound physiological effect on the human brain. These technological advancements demonstrate how a child's exposure to trauma can dramatically transform the physiological structure of the brain, thereby impacting their physical and emotional development and long-term health. Positive stress is the body's normal response to danger or other challenging events such as the first day of school, moving to a new neighborhood, or a reaction to a thunderstorm. In a safe and nurturing family environment, the child will learn to regulate what is referred to as tolerable stress.[57]

Unlike positive stress, toxic stress occurs when a threat is repeated to the point where the child's body is producing an overload of stress hormones such as cortisol and adrenaline. According to Drs. Ted R. Miller (Pacific Institute of Research and Evaluation) and Nancy N. Carlson (Walden University College of Social and Behavioral Health) in their publication *Adverse Childhood Experiences: Responding to a Cross-Generational Opioid Tragedy,* "Untreated stress leads to internalizing and externalizing disorders, smoking, obesity, and drug and alcohol problems. Critically, it can permanently change brain structure and function. . . ACEs exposure is a common gateway to opioid use problems. It is associated with roughly triple the odds that children and adults will misuse opioids."[58]

Traumatic events and experiences can occur in the home, in the community, and from the environment.[59] Chronic toxic stress, regardless of the source of the traumatic event, can adversely affect the child's ability to respond to these events with resilience. But like ACEs, resilience can be built in the home and in the community.

ACEs in the Home

Think for a moment about situations where frequent violence exists in the home or where a child experiences abuse on a regular basis. Chronic toxic stress occurs when the child is living in a condition of red alert mode for months or years at a time. Without protective factors to regulate the child's reaction to the threat, these stress hormones can alter the brain.

Conversely, a healthy home environment where children are connected, nurtured, and attended to counters many of the risk factors associated with ACEs. Protective factors include a wide range of relationships and environments that build resilience against toxic stress and can result in a slow healing of the stress-induced damages from chronic toxic stress. The CDC cites the following individual and family protective factors that can reduce the impact of adverse childhood experiences or prevent them from occurring in the first place. These include safe and stable family structure, friendships, schools, and caring adults outside of the family.[60]

Since school is the environment where kids spend the bulk of their time outside of the home, teachers and administrators play a vital role in the detection of trauma in the home. Trauma-informed education and programming are therefore becoming foundations for educators and school administrators as they change their approach in the classroom and in the schoolyard. When asked how you read a child's presenting demeanor at school when you suspect something is off, or not quite right, Lara Merchant, early childhood special educator for the city of Barre, Vermont, responded:

"It's really important to build a relationship with a child. If a child becomes dysregulated and possibly violent, then that's not the time to try to correct their behavior. It's not the time to rationalize and try to have a conversation with them. When dysregulated, they're way back in their reptilian brain and their prefrontal cortex is offline. They are not logically thinking in that moment. I believe in connecting before correcting. So you could say, 'You look like you're really mad', or use body-based language such as, 'I'm seeing you're really tense, and your body seems tight right now.' Then just leave it and see if they say anything. Once that connection happens, that's when things can start to de-escalate."[61]

I asked about the importance of trauma-informed approaches in the classroom. Merchant said, "When schools invite behavior specialists to come into the classroom to handle more extreme behaviors, who don't even know the student, that doesn't work. Why is this student going to want to listen to them and respond to them? Especially if they have a trauma history; they're not going to trust somebody they don't know. For a behavior specialist to come into the classroom to try to correct the behavior is an antiquated system, which is what many schools do. So that's why teachers and support staff have to be trauma-informed: because they're the ones who are building the relationships with the students. They have to be the ones to support their students."

ACEs in the Community

In addition to individual experiences and family risk factors for children, the community where we live can also lead to risk factors for childhood trauma. Discrimination, social injustice, and poverty are among the root causes for community-based adverse childhood experiences. Crime, unemployment, easy access to drugs, and homelessness are other examples. Events like the 2023 shootings in Lewiston or the opioid epidemic in many communities across the United States are specific examples.

Adverse community environments lead to lack of trust and social cohesion within the community, leaving residents feeling disempowered. Lack of housing and reliable access to food leads to hopelessness. Community resilience suffers if intentional efforts are not made to withstand existing and future community harm. It follows, therefore, that individual and family resilience are also adversely impacted in the face of community crisis.

Similar to individual and family protective factors, a community can help mitigate the impact of childhood trauma through community action, economic vitality, and access to healthcare, housing, and safe places to play.[62]

The good news is that a coordinated community effort to address these socioeconomic issues helps to provide individuals with the support they need in difficult times. Creating community conditions that enhance residents' well-being is a critical component of building community resilience; however, service delivery differs in scope and priority depending on the provider or community-based organization offering that service. This is why a *trauma-informed*, coordinated approach to building community resilience is so important.

Human connection and meaningful relationships help build community resilience against tragic events in the community. In his book *Fragile Neighborhoods*, which talks about structures that can strengthen the community, author Seth Kaplan wrote:

"It's community structures that connect. These can be anything from schools to coffee shops to churches to kinship ties to public institutions. One way to measure the success or the health of a place is to look at the quality and quantity of its place-specific institutions—economic, social, religious, cultural, civic, whatever, If they're specific to a place, they are likely connecting people there. For example, a local coffee shop—whether it has one or three locations—is much more likely to care about a place and connect people there than a national chain. It is also important to differentiate between friends and relationships. We have at best a small number of friends, but what really matters is our relationships of trust and support. While there has been a decline in friends, the decline in relationships of this nature has been far more dramatic and significant. Moreover, a lot of these friendships have become much more transactional in nature. I think the fewer trusting, supportive relationships you have, the fewer real friendships you have, and the fewer people you can depend on and share time with, and this leads to a great weakening in the social glue within any community."[63]

ACEs in the Environment

Natural disasters such as earthquakes, hurricanes, and blizzards affect the community and the families who live there. These natural disasters and other environmental events, including the COVID pandemic and the impact of climate change, can also create an existential threat to a community. Witness the devastating impact of Hurricane Helene to the southeast United States in early fall 2024.

The COVID-19 pandemic had a devastating impact in terms of death, hospitalizations, and quarantines, which led to fear and isolation, which in turn led to depression and anxiety. Our children were especially impacted due to the loss of social interactions with friends and the necessary reliance on e-learning to connect to the classroom.

During the pandemic, the United States saw significant increases in alcohol, drug, and suicide deaths in 2020 and 2021. The CDC also found that there was a rise in alcohol-induced mortality from 2019 to 2020 (10.4 to 13.1 deaths per 100,000 people, respectively), and that increased consumption during the height of the pandemic was largely due to related stress, loneliness, and social isolation.[64]

We've seen that adverse childhood experiences, whether experienced in the home, the community, or as a result of a global environmental event, can lead to behavioral and/or health issues for individuals. We've also seen that there is a predictability of the impact of trauma on populations. The good news is that what is predictable is also preventable.

CHAPTER 3

TRAUMA INTERRUPTED

Positive Childhood Experiences

Just as adverse childhood experiences have a negative effect on individuals, families, and communities, positive childhood experiences (PCEs) can buffer against the health effects of adverse experiences for individuals, families, and communities. Dr. Christina Bethell, professor of public health at Johns Hopkins University, has conducted extensive research on the effects of positive childhood experiences (PCEs), and provides a roadmap to help our children build resilience and flourish as adults.

According to Dr. Bethell, assessing and proactively promoting PCEs may reduce adult mental and relational health problems, even in the concurrent presence of ACEs.[65] Dr. Bethell analyzed the data from the 2019 Wisconsin Behavioral Risk Factor Study of a representative sample of 6,188 adults eighteen and older in that state. In this survey, respondents were asked how often they:

1. Felt able to talk to their family about feelings

2. Felt their family stood by them during difficult times

3. Enjoyed participating in community traditions

4. Felt a sense of belonging in high school

5. Felt supported by friends

6. Had at least two non-parent adults who took genuine interest in them

7. Felt safe and protected by an adult in their home

From this survey, Dr. Bethell found that adults with fewer PCEs (0-2) were over five times more likely to experience depression and poor mental health compared to adults who had a high number PCEs (6-7).[66]

A similar study published by the National Library of Health found PCEs involving children who had supportive relationships and nurturing environments are strongly associated with improved mental and physical health in adulthood.[67] Survey participants who reported having strong peer relationships during childhood, had supportive school environments, and lived in neighborhoods where they felt safe, were less likely to report health problems as adults.

As with predictability of health issues in adults as a result of ACEs, there is now a correlation between PCEs and improved health in adults. This correlation means that interventions in the home and in the community can have a role in building resilience in our children to withstand challenges as adults. We now know that adverse childhood experiences contribute to toxic stress, which has been shown to lead to poor health outcomes when left unmitigated. We also know that positive childhood experiences protect against and are likely to disrupt the harmful health effects of toxic stress to promote healing and build resilience, leading to improved health outcomes.

In October 2020, I attended a full-day workshop with Dr. Bethell where she introduced the concept of building community ecosystems to help develop flourishing adolescents. The purpose of the workshop was to educate my fellow ACEs master trainers and me with the knowledge and tools to help our communities develop interventions against adverse childhood experiences. It was here that I began to fully understand the impact of ACEs, and that by delivering the restorative benefits of PCEs, we as communities can begin to break the trans-generational cycle of trauma. PCEs block toxic stress and promote healing. Positive childhood experiences lead to resilience. Resilience leads to healthy outcomes. Through prevention programs the community experience can then become a primary source of interventions that ultimately lead to healthy individuals and families.

The community plays a vital role in providing positive experiences to its youth. A single interaction with a child can change their life for the better, and there are countless opportunities for members of the community to interact. We typically think of recreational organizations such as youth sports, YMCA, the arts, and other club-oriented programs. However, neighbors, childcare providers, social services staff, teachers, mentors, tutors, businesses, law enforcement, first responders, and court advocates are other examples of parties that often come in contact with our youth.

Social Determinants of Health

Social determinants of health are the social, economic, physical, and other conditions that affect a range of health outcomes for a community. For example, a community's quality of life is affected by providing access to basic resources including housing, education, public safety, and healthy food. The US Department of Health and Human Services, in their Healthy People 2030 initiative, defines a community's social determinants of health across five categories—employment, early education development and education, access to health services, access to a healthy diet, and civic participation—that affect a wide range of health, functioning, and quality-of-life outcomes and risks.[68]

As you can imagine, there are ample examples of disparities and inequalities in terms of access to social determinants of health. Poverty, racism, social status, criminal background, and sexuality are only a handful of biases facing members of the community, which in turn create barriers to healthy outcomes for marginalized individuals. For example, in the addiction recovery space, individuals with justice involvement have profound barriers when re-entering the community, especially when housing or employment are sought. Recovery Ready Communities provide justice-involved individuals with the capacity to overcome these barriers.

CHAPTER 4

RESILIENCE

In his book *Community: The Structure of Belonging*, author Peter Block introduces the concept of a restorative community. He states, "Restoration comes from the choice to value possibility and relatedness over problems, needs, self-interest, and the rest of the stuck community's agenda. Restoration is created by the kinds of conversations we initiate with each other. These conversations are the leverage point for an alternative future."[69]

Applying this concept to communities in crisis due to the impact of addiction, a restorative or resilient community can be thought of as one with a common view of relationships, purpose, and accountability to address addiction. The resilient community rises to the challenge of addressing the root causes of addiction, and provides a roadmap to prevention, recovery, and treatment services for its citizens.

Building resilient communities is essential to improving public health, safety, and economic well-being for the individuals and families who live and work there. Communities can also be a source of healing in the face of crisis. Further, resilient communities can be a source of protective factors that keep us safe should a crisis occur.

Where does community begin? As soon as we step outside of our home.

The Concept of Connective Tissue in the Community

In the medical field, connective tissue is defined as tissue that supports, protects, and gives structure to other tissues and organs in the body. This definition can also be applied to organizations and communities.

I recently attended a 12-step meeting where the guest speaker used the term "connective tissue" as the bond that binds together members of the Alcoholics Anonymous community. His point was that we in the AA program share a common understanding of each other's recovery journey, but more importantly, we have a shared common goal of sobriety for our members, and especially the so-called "newcomer."

One of the frequently repeated mantras in the recovery community is that the opposite of addiction is connection. Where do we make connections? In communities. Why do we seek these connections? Affiliation and security. According to Mental Health

America, a leading nonprofit dedicated to the advancement of mental health, "creating and sustaining a community around you is important to your mental health. Humans are social creatures, meaning our brains are wired to seek connection with others. These connections allow us to share interests and feel a sense of belonging and security."[70]

Members of communities have attached themselves to causes for ages. Fraternal organizations such as the Knights of Columbus, Rotary, Lions Club, and many other similar groups have sprung up in cities across the country. Youth sports, arts, civic organizations, and social clubs are only a few examples of formal organizations that bring people together, often serving the needs of the community. These are examples of what I refer to as *connective tissue* within the community.

Communities often come together in times of needs. Perhaps the most recent and obvious example is the COVID-19 pandemic. Certainly, mental health, addiction, and the opioid epidemic in particular qualify as causes that bring members of the community together. But of what value is connection if it is so ingrained in the community's history and culture that it fails to adapt to changes? To what degree does the community have the resiliency to navigate through and respond to such issues when history and culture prevent it from meeting the needs of today?

Resilience is defined as the capacity to withstand or to recover quickly from difficulties. NAMI applies this definition to individuals: "Resiliency reduces the harmful effects of stress and trauma, acting as a buffer to help you maintain your well-being. Strengthening and adding protective factors, like social support, access to resources, and caring for your physical health, all serve to help you effectively counteract cumulative stress."[71]

The same concept applies to the community. Community resilience is a measure of the sustained ability of a community to utilize available resources to respond to, withstand, and recover from adverse situations. Although this often refers to disasters such as floods, tornados, earthquakes, war, pandemics, and famine, community resilience also applies to public health crises such as mental health and addiction. In the case of the addiction, protective factors can include prevention, treatment, harm reduction, and recovery support.

According to Tamarack Institute, a global community engagement consultancy based in Waterloo, Ontario, Canada, resilience is a "collaboration's effort to increase its capacity to bounce back from setbacks, mobilize around emerging opportunities, take time to reflect, and be prepared for future challenges. In these days of rapid change and disruption, resilience—the ability to adapt to emerging opportunities and respond to unanticipated challenges is an essential capacity. Resilience is about building a collaboration's capacity to shift, adapt, and change, and is also focused on the overall health and well-being of the collaboration and the community."[72]

From author Seth Kaplan: "Each of us is embedded in circles of relationships and institutions that shape everything from our psychology and beliefs to how we treat each other and what life choices we have and make.[73] . . . Real community produces an eco-system in which every member is deeply embedded, not a collection of relationships that can be picked up and moved if the owners so desire it."[74]

What is a Resilient Community?

At 6:56 p.m. on October 25, 2023, a lone gunman entered Just-In-Time Recreation, a bowling alley in Lewiston, Maine, and opened fire on staff and patrons. Twelve minutes later, while law enforcement and first responders rushed to that location, the same shooter walked into Schemengees Bar and Grille, about four miles away from Just-In-Time, also in Lewiston and opened fire on staff and patrons of that business. In total, eighteen people died and another thirteen suffered injuries. Of all the senseless mass shootings over the decades here in the United States, this incident hit especially close to home as at that time I was working with leaders of Auburn and Lewiston, communities who were taking early steps of building a recovery ready community. At the time, I was the statewide director of the Maine Recovery Friendly Workplace (RFW) program, and I had been meeting with several businesses for RFW orientation in the days prior to the shootings.

In the hours, days, and weeks following the discovery of the shooter who had ultimately taken his own life, a swarm of local, county, state, and federal agencies converged on Lewiston to establish public safety, coordinate communications across numerous agencies, conduct reunification of residents and family members who survived the attack, provide family assistance, and establish a community resilience center.

A few months after the shooting, Danielle Parent, JD, LCSW, who was named director of the Maine Resiliency Center, accepted my invitation to speak at the annual Pinetree Institute Resilience Conference, which was focused on the subject of community resilience. The title of her presentation was "Building Community Resilience After Mass Violence."[75] There are several lessons to be learned from her talk that directly apply to any community seeking to build resilience against adverse scenario, including addiction.

"Where to start?" was Danielle's opening rhetorical question to the conference attendees. "If you were asked to support a community in rebuilding resiliency in the wake of mass trauma, where would you start?" These are the lessons she shared:

1. **Know your community.** Know your people, history, businesses, resources, needs, values, culture, dynamics, connection, and disconnection. Every community is different. One notable fact about the culture of Lewiston is that it is one of the most ethnically diverse communities in the United States with open arms extended to immigrants, refugees, and asylum seekers from several parts of the

world, including Somalia, Haiti, Afghanistan, and Ukraine. Language and culture matters in Lewiston.

2. **Understand the impact.** Where do the "ripples" flow to? Where are the boulders?

3. **Know who is impacted.** The list is exhaustive: victims, survivors, family, friends, loved ones, first responders, businesses, victim advocates, providers, and extended community. All were traumatized by the event.

4. **Know the impacts of the trauma.** The impact is different for everyone. Grief, anger, sadness, fear, numbness, dissociation, anxiety, and many, many reactions can be experienced by individuals and the community.

5. **Provide support.** Create safe spaces. Provide meaningful access to support services. The approach to support in Lewiston was to create a low-barrier community safe space that could rapidly adapt to the unique needs of visitors seeking services.

6. **Prepare for challenges.** In the case of the Lewiston tragedy, challenges included eligibility for benefits, access to and sharing of information, dealing with the media and the press, cultural sensitivity, funding, scheduling, predicting the needs, volunteer and donor management, logistics, dealing with criticism, and self-care.

What was the "secret sauce" that led to the resource center's positive impact on the community? Connection.

Trauma-Informed Community Engagement

Resilient communities are both prepared for traumatic events and have capacity to address such events in their aftermath. It is logical then that resilient communities utilize trauma-informed approaches to engagement. Once again we can learn from the response to the tragedy in Lewiston:[76]

- Trauma impacts everyone differently
- Traumatic grief is complex
- The words we choose are important
- We could all use a little more grace
- We don't always take good care of one another
- We have the capacity for greatness through community

- Community and connection are foundational to resiliency

- There is an impact on providers

- Be prepared that it will change you

Without ignoring or minimizing the trauma experienced by individuals, families, and the community itself, the effective engagement model should help to build a path to new opportunities, relationships, connections, and important life moments.

What do we mean by "trauma-informed?" The CDC defines six principles of a Trauma-Informed Approach to community building:[77]

1. **Safety:** the community prevents violence across the lifespan and creates safe physical environments.

2. **Trustworthiness:** the community fosters positive relationships among residents, city hall, law enforcement, schools, and others.

3. **Empowerment:** the community ensures opportunities for growth are available to all.

4. **Collaboration:** the community promotes involvement of residents and partnerships among agencies.

5. **Peer Support:** the community engages residents to work together on issues of common concern.

6. **History, Gender, Culture:** the community values and supports history, culture, and diversity.

Trauma-informed care shifts the conversation from "What is wrong with you?" to "What happened to you?" According to the Center for Health Care Strategies, trauma-informed care seeks to:

- Realize the widespread impact of trauma and understands paths to recovery

- Recognize the signs and symptoms of trauma in patients, families, and staff

- Integrate knowledge about trauma into policies, procedures, and practices

- Actively avoids re-traumatization[78]

Molly Louison-Semrow, associate director at Pinetree Institute, shared her take on being trauma-informed and the value of applying that in coalition environments. "If you're working with human beings, you're doing trauma work. It's not about specializing in trauma, it's about an understanding that we should assume that the people that we're centering in our work, and the people that we're interacting with, very likely have a trauma history."[79]

Putting trauma-informed community engagement into practice requires creating a safe environment for members to participate without causing secondary trauma. Staffing of professionals who are educated in trauma-informed practices can raise the capacity for trauma-informed services and practices. Although skilled leadership is critical, it is equally important to welcome and involve community members to participate in the planning process for the coalition. Finally, open communication, active listening, and documentation of the process and results will ensure transparency.

Example: Trauma Responsive Monadnock

The Monadnock region of southwestern New Hampshire has embarked on a journey to bring trauma-informed perspective to the region and formed a coalition to address trauma in the community. The coalition applied for and received a three-year grant from the New Hampshire Children's Health Foundation that allowed for the hiring of a project manager to build the capacity for Trauma Responsive Monadnock (TRM). While the initiative is focused on interventions to prevent and mitigate trauma in youth, it works with people across the lifespan—since youth caregivers need to be trauma-informed if the cycles of intergenerational trauma are to be interrupted.

That project manager, Anena Hansen, began in April 2023 by talking with dozens of people around the Monadnock region, from law enforcement to social service providers, from town officials to health care professionals, asking them what they saw as the greatest trauma-related needs and what solutions they wished for. Over time, various themes arose, and the TRM coalition—comprising a couple dozen community members, from mental health providers to county employees to retirees—used that feedback to create a two-year strategic plan. With the broad objective of creating the Monadnock region as a trauma-informed community, they set the specific goals of educating community members on trauma, enrolling community leaders to implement policy changes within their spheres of influence, creating a digital database of trauma-related professionals and programming through the region, and establishing a series of "youth support cohorts" to connect professionals in all sectors who work with youth experiencing trauma.

I first met Hansen at Pinetree Institute's fourth Annual Resilience Conference in May 2023 in Eliot, Maine. We caught up recently for a discussion on her coalition's progress. "The big thing that we're working on right now is creating awareness of the impact of trauma on our children. To start making an impact, we've been primarily focused on promoting more collaboration in the professional sphere—taking the resources that already exist and putting them together in new ways. The capacity is there for that. So I'm a convener in a lot of ways, a connector, because we have a foundation of good resources, and we're just building on that."[80]

One of the immediate challenges presented to Hansen is the size and diversity of the Monadnock region. She explained, "We have thirty-three towns in our catchment area, the Greater Monadnock Public Health Network, with a total population of about 110,000 people. We're slowly working to bring together all the educators, guidance counselors, and school administrators—basically everyone who is interacting with kids at school—as well as DCYF [the New Hampshire Division for Children, Youth and Families], the homeless shelter, the community kitchen, mental health providers, all the social service agencies, and first responders. Basically anybody who, in their professional capacity, interacts with youth who are experiencing or have experienced trauma, whether acute or chronic."

What struck me during the conversation was that Hansen and the Trauma Responsive Monadnock coalition were doing precisely the same thing that we in Portsmouth had done three or four years earlier. We too started with a grassroots effort to start the conversation and to assess our initial priorities. Hansen continued, "We started our youth support cohorts by organizing town-specific meetings where professionals came together to exchange contacts and explain the services they offer, so that they all know where to refer families who are facing different kinds of trauma. The very first one we had, in June (2024), was held in our county seat and attended by thirty-three people, all the way up to the county commissioner. We started the conversation with what was missing, what are the quick wins that we could do something about right now, and what are some long term goals towards which we could work."

That town, Keene, has the largest population of the GMPHN, with about twenty-five thousand people. The next largest town, Peterborough, has only sixty-five hundred people, but their initial youth support cohort meeting landed on roughly the same needs: better communication between law enforcement and first responders and schools and direct youth service providers. Keene's self-identified interventions look different than Peterborough's, however, and such will presumably be the case with the smaller cohorts, which are expected to form by school districts since there are so few individual resources at the town-specific level.

Other trauma-targeted interventions underway include a free "Trauma-Informed Service" training available to any business or organization. TIS is a two-hour workshop that teaches the basics of trauma, how it shows up, and how to mitigate its negative impact. In the first three months, seven free trainings were attended by nearly a hundred representatives of for-profit and nonprofit entities around the region. From here, community leaders were targeted to begin the process of implementing policy-level changes in their organization.

The trauma-focused professional database also launched online to support youth cohort participants to connect with ease, and content creation is underway for a broad social media campaign that will be featured on dozens of regional social media accounts, from schools to businesses to police departments, in order to ensure that as many people as possible are exposed to the basics of trauma awareness in bite-sized pieces.

Trauma Responsive Monadnock continues to expand, pivoting whenever possible to respond to specific needs. In the wake of several youth deaths by accident and suicide, they are currently developing community trauma response protocols that clarify chains of command and the role to be played by professionals and volunteers who offer any form of support for acute trauma. As a coalition, TRM leans into each need as it arises, working together to make the Monadnock region of New Hampshire a safe, connected community for all.

CHAPTER 5

UNDERSTANDING RECOVERY

Individual Recovery

SAMHSA defines recovery as "a process of change through which individuals improve their health and wellness, live self-directed lives, and strive to reach their full potential."[81] This is a content-rich sentence that can be broken down into three very important stand-alone parts.

1. *A process of change* connotes that the path to recovery is just that—a journey. There is no destination. Initiating the process of change at its core represents change. A person in recovery from alcoholism or addiction, or a person with other chronic illnesses such as heart disease or diabetes, goes through a similar process of change whereby they make a conscious decision to make life changes.

2. *Live self-directed lives* requires the individual to take responsibility for their recovery, to take ownership and define their path to recovery.

3. *Strive to meet their full potential* sets an aspirational end-state that is self-defined.

Full potential goes well beyond one's career or socioeconomic status. It is intentionally ambiguous. It can mean physical, mental, or spiritual health. It could mean financial prosperity, or it could simply mean happiness. The word "strive" tells us that the outcome is not necessarily guaranteed. That there is effort involved. Setbacks are likely and must be overcome to reach that potential.

When I entered treatment in 2012 for alcohol and substance use, I had no clue about these concepts. All I knew was that I was done. Toast. I had had enough. But I did not know how to get better on my own, which is the entire point of this book. A person entering treatment or any path to recovery is unlikely to know how to get help on their own. Which is where family and community enters the mix.

Family Recovery

Because addiction is a family disease, family recovery programming is often sought. Although there are increasing community-based organizations and providers offering services, it is sometimes difficult to find. Some of the challenges facing family members include confusion, stigma, sadness, anxiety, isolation, and knowing where to call to get help. In my experience, organizations such as NAMI or peer-based family recovery programming at a recovery community center are a great place to start.

One of the primary barriers to families seeking recovery services is stigma. Many families are afraid to seek recovery services out of fear of being stigmatized. No one wants to announce to the world that their child, spouse, parent, or significant other is struggling with addiction. Overcoming that fear is often the first step for the family to get recovery help.

In their publication *The Ripple Effect: The Impact of the Opioid Epidemic on Children and Families,* authors Suzanne D. Brundage and Carol Levine break down the impact of addiction to family members and provide a framework for communities to support these families. Included in this framework are suggestions that in order to reduce stigma, the community should "promote nonjudgmental language" and "develop education programs on the nature of SUD and its treatment."[82]

Most SUD treatment centers offer "Family Day" or other similar programming that provides education and supportive services to a resident's family. However, it is important for the family members to feel "heard" by the treatment staff, as members of the family are dealing with their own trauma. Many are still raw and feeling angry with their loved one.

In my case, in 2012 while I was a patient at Michael's House in Palm Springs, initially my wife had little interest in attending any family programming. "It's his problem and his fault. This is not about me," she claimed. Only through the very skillful listening sessions between my wife and the center's clinicians did she finally accept that she, as an affected other, and we as a couple, could benefit from this important event.

Community Recovery

As mentioned in the prior chapter, it is said in the circles of recovery that addiction is the opposite of connection. An addictive mind craves isolation where secrets are believed to be safe. Our underlying issues, whether they are trauma, fear, anxiety, or hopelessness, operate best when the addict is alone and left to their thoughts. The isolated mind can be a very scary place. A healthy community can and should provide residents with this ability to connect and build relationships.

In the face of the national opioid epidemic, communities also have an opportunity to lead. Addiction has a devastating social impact on communities, affecting public health, safety, and social welfare. Cities and towns across the country have initiated government-driven or grassroots efforts to build resilience against this epidemic.

Author Peter Block, in his book *Community: The Structure of Belonging,* suggests that the opposite of isolation is belonging. "To belong is to be related to and a part of something. It is membership, the experience of being at home in the broadest sense of the phrase . . . to belong to a community is to act as a creator and co-owner of that community."[83] In other words, members of a connected community have skin in the game. They have a vested interest in the health of the community.

Connection requires a reciprocal relationship with a person, group of people, or with members and institutions of the community. Connection to another person suggests both parties have made an implicit social contract. I have found this especially true with communities. Among many other examples, a community can be a city or town, a club, a self-help organization, or an informal gathering of friends around a common purpose.

As Kaplan writes in his book *Fragile Neighborhoods,* "neighborhoods rich with social capital not only reduce everyday stress, but also offer higher-quality institutions and networks: the kind of resources residents can call upon in the future if they need help. . . ."[84]

As a child growing up in Leominster, Massachusetts, a diverse blue-collar factory town in the north-central part of the state, I benefited greatly from the gifts of a close-knit community of ethnic neighborhoods. In my book *A Place in Time: Youth, Community & Baseball,* the fundamental theme is the power of the neighborhood as community. The original intent for that book was simply to celebrate the fiftieth anniversary of a spectacular consecutive three-year run of championships for our city's Babe Ruth All-Stars teams. What I found from the research and the interviews I conducted led me to the conclusion that this story was about so much more.

That story was indeed about the players and coaches, but it was perhaps most importantly a story about the role of the community, its neighborhoods, and school-yards where kids had safe places and opportunities to thrive. It was about sports and other recreational activities that provided us with the opportunity to develop the necessary skills to cope and succeed as adults. But sadly, that story was also about the erosion of those very things at a time when we as a society perhaps need them most.[85] On countless playgrounds, sandlots, parking lots, school athletic fields and neighborhoods, hundreds of us kids developed an interest in, developed the skills for, and sustained a passion for the game of baseball. Volunteers groomed the fields, sold the concessions, raised the money, and coached the teams. Parents, relatives, neighbors, and complete strangers showed up to watch us play. Newspapers sent reporters to cover our games. Local community radio stations covered our games with live broadcasts. We, the players, were a reflection of the community.

The community, just like the individual and the family, can be "the patient." How does the community recover from the impact of addiction? We now shift our focus to a solution.

SECTION 2

A SOLUTION

CHAPTER 6

THE COMMUNITY AS THE PATIENT

Many of us have received SUD treatment and recovery services as a patient. Others of us have benefited from family recovery programs. But what happens when the community becomes the patient? What does a community do when public safety, public health, and its economy are impacted from addiction?

A community has an obligation to protect its citizens from crisis. Cities and towns have the responsibility for public health and safety. But what about the health of the community itself? As the Recovery Research Institute proposes, "Over time, when hopelessness and learned helplessness become ingrained in community culture and transmitted across generations, the community itself is in need of recovery from alcohol and other drug problems."[86]

SAMHSA defines community recovery as a "voluntary process through which a community uses the assertive resolution of alcohol and other drug-related problems as a vehicle for collective healing, community renewal, and enhanced inter-generational resilience. A compassionate response in a recovery-ready community will greatly reduce the social, economic, and health burden of substance use disorders on the community level."[87]

Community engagement brings together the skills, knowledge, and experiences of diverse groups to create and/or implement solutions that work for all members of the community.[88] In the case of community engagement, community stakeholders may include:

- Businesses

- Chambers of Commerce

- Community-based organizations

- Faith-based organizations

- First responders

- Fraternal organizations

- Healthcare and hospitals

- Local government and departments

- Media

- Parents, family members

- People in recovery

- People who use drugs

- People with justice involvement history

- Philanthropic community

- Providers

- Public safety and law enforcement

- Schools and administrators

- State government representatives

- Treatment centers

- Youth

Brown et al. propose a recovery-specific community engagement framework with the following stakeholders[89]:

- Recovery-informed institutional services

- Recovery community centers

- Collegiate recovery programs

- Recovery/drug courts

- Mutual-aid organizations

- Recovery community organizations

- Prevention organizations

- Peer recovery services

- Harm reduction organizations

- Re-entry services organizations

- Recovery residences

- Medical treatment services

- Advocacy organizations

- Recovery high schools

We will learn about the approaches of recovery-ready communities and their heroic efforts to save and improve the lives of their citizens. Before we dive into the solution, let us first shed a light on the concept and value of recovery capital.

CHAPTER 7

BUILDING RECOVERY CAPITAL

What is Recovery Capital?

According to author and researcher William White, "Recovery capital is conceptually linked to natural recovery, solution-focused therapy, strengths-based case management, recovery management, resilience and protective factors, and the ideas of hardiness, wellness, and global health."[90] Putting this concept into practice, recovery capital can be thought of as the sum of recovery assets within an individual or a community.

Author Alison Jones Webb writes that "as a community, we can create physical, cultural, and social environments that are conducive to sustained recovery," and that "creating recovery capital is the most important activity that we can do to help people in recovery and their families heal and move ahead in their lives."[91]

When thinking about creating capacity in the community, the Recovery-Oriented Systems of Care (ROSC) model suggests that recovery capital is "coordinated community-based services that are person-centered and build strength and resilience of individuals, families, and communities."[92] With the ROSC framework in mind, recovery capital is created when "internal and external resources can be drawn upon to pursue, achieve, sustain, and enhance a life of recovery or well-being."[93]

I like to think of it as the amount of water in a glass. The more water in the glass, the greater the amount of recovery capital.

Increasingly, recovery capital is becoming a term identified and linked to recovery-ready communities:[94]

- **Personal recovery capital:** Examples include self-awareness, self-regulation, resilience, coping skills, and basic human needs such as shelter, food, and security.

- **Family/social recovery capital:** When thinking of social capital, think of connection, relationships, bridging, and social engagement.

- **Community recovery capital:** Examples include treatment, recovery support, and response to the individual's basic needs of shelter, food, and security.

While recovery capital indeed helps improve coping strategies and enhance the quality of life for those in long-term recovery from mental health disorders and SUD, we must be mindful that recovery capital is wasted unless *all* of those in need have access to this capital. This includes access for marginalized populations within the community.

Access to recovery capital does not require abstinence on the part of the individual. Like other chronic illnesses, individuals with a substance use disorder may experience setbacks. Would we deny a person with heart disease access to housing or food if they suffered another heart attack?

Dr. Alex Elswick, a member of the faculty at the University of Kentucky, suggests that recovery capital extends well beyond the traditional treatment and recovery continuum of care, and that basic human needs (housing, food, water, rest) and safety needs must be met before an individual can realistically be expected to enter the system of care for SUD.[95] "Should we wait for individuals to become abstinent before building recovery capital? Should abstinence be a pre-condition for housing, social services, caregiving, mental health services, continued treatment, or acceptance in the recovery community?" he asks rhetorically. "We don't expect individuals with other chronic illness to be abstinent from their illnesses."

Example: Measuring Recovery Capital

How do we measure recovery capital? How do we measure a community's capacity for resilience? David Whitesock is the founder and CEO of Commonly Well, PBC, a company that helps service providers, investors, and policy-makers gain client visibility, insight, and predictive capabilities through the use of a survey tool referred to as the Recovery Capacity Index (RCI).[96] Whitesock suggests that community resilience is "the capacity for communities to withstand an impact, a disturbance, and bounce back to the status quo."[97]

Measuring recovery capacity is an iterative process beginning with an initial assessment, review of the initial results, a refining of the assessment criteria, conducting a follow-on assessment, analysis of the results, acting on the conclusions from the analysis, and repeat as necessary to achieve desired outcomes.

I asked Whitesock about the best way to get started.

"I would have the coalition do a RCI in that session," he said. "When they walk in the door, before the meeting even begins, we make it very clear that we're going to ask them to take five to ten minutes, and they are going to complete this questionnaire. My suggestion, and this is based on my experience, if I were to be in that room with the coalition members, I would ask, 'What does this coalition want to learn. What are the outcomes? Where do we want to focus? What data can we capture?' I would suggest that it's going to be the community that's going to give us that observation. At some point before the end of that meeting we put the data up on the wall and show them the RCI. That would be the initial measurement of recovery capital in the community. This process is more formalized as the coalition evolves."

What do we do with that data?

"The next exercise is the part where we conduct analytics including dashboards that are relevant to the coalition's needs. As the data is coming in, we create and share as preliminary results. It's not scrubbed yet, it's just quick analysis. If the coalition needs to adjust, now's the time to do it. As opposed to waiting five years to get to the end. And the benefits of having a system for measuring the coalition's work are better decision making, the ability to make course corrections, setting priorities, increasing focus, and perhaps most importantly, creating accountability for the coalition."[98]

CHAPTER 8

BUILDING THE COALITION

Why Form a Coalition?

Coalition building is a common approach to community engagement. Coalitions are effective because they can accomplish what would be difficult for an individual or single organization to accomplish alone. The value of a coalition approach to community engagement is that it creates new collective resources and connects people to them. Each coalition member brings their own network of connections to the group, therefore creating a larger network for deploying resources and ultimately effecting change.

I first met Lisa Attygalle, director of community engagement at Tamarack Institute, in 2022 when I was invited to participate in a community coalition for the Lewiston-Auburn region of Maine. According to Attygalle, Tamarack's view is that when considering a coalition to address large-scale community needs, a systems infrastructure or "backbone" needs to exist.

"Everyone can have the best intentions of collaborating or working differently, but unless you have the people and the structures to hold it—to care about the process, to care about who's part of decision making, to help resources flow equitably, to care about sustainability of initiatives, to define outcomes and measure those outcomes—those intentions may fall short. This backbone provides shared leadership and accountability."[99]

In order to develop community interest around the coalition, there needs to be a sense of urgency around the issue behind the coalition. Examples include climate change, violent crime, or in this book's case, addiction. If there is no urgency around an issue, it will be difficult getting potential members to the table, to get funding to support the coalition, and to sustain commitment from coalition members once the coalition is operational.

According to Attygalle, "Oftentimes a coalition comes together because you want to change how the current system works. The work could be to change a policy, to innovate and create a better way of doing things, to fill a gap, to change mindsets, or to build capacity. The work is sustainable when we embed these changes into existing structures so that it becomes the new normal."

Tamarack Institute uses the Collective Impact model, where there are three pre-conditions that must exist for long-term success when initiating a collaborative (coalition):

1. **An Influential Champion:** An individual or small group who commands the respect necessary to bring senior-level cross-sector leaders together and keep them actively engaged over time.

2. **Adequate Financial Resourcing:** Adequate financial resources to last at least two to three years and generally involving at least one anchor funder to support needed infrastructure and planning.

3. **A Sense of Urgency for Change:** A new opportunity or crisis that convinces people that a particular issue must be acted upon now and/or that a new approach is needed.[100]

A Framework for Coalition Building

An important first step in building a community coalition is to bring together a small group of "founding members" to act as an ad hoc steering committee. The steering committee will lay the foundation for future coalition work such as assessing community needs, recruiting coalition members, orienting members to the mission and best practices, and developing the operating framework of the coalition. SAMHSA provides a framework and useful guidance for coalition building.[101]

1. Understanding Your Community
2. Identify Potential Coalition Members
3. Orient Members to SUD and Evidence-Based Practices
4. Develop Coalition Rules of Engagement

Understanding Your Community

In this step we invite representative members of the community to come forth and define the needs of the populations to be served. Many coalitions, such as the Greater Portsmouth Recovery Coalition, conduct initial research without yet having formed a formal coalition. In other cases, such as the Strafford County Addiction Task Force, they utilize assessment data from other sources such as the Community Health Needs Assessment (CHNA) conducted by Wentworth-Douglass Hospital. The objective is to get an initial sense of the priorities going forward, not necessarily to the exclusion of other issues, but to triage the data for initial focus and action. Needs assessment can be quantitative or qualitative. Avoid overthinking the process of setting initial priorities.

Ashley Wheeler, manager at Strafford County Public Health Network, and coordinator of the Strafford County Addiction Task Force, explains the process of setting priorities: "We took the priorities back to our work groups or convened stakeholders that were experts in that area, or that work in that area, or informed in this work. We took it back to our Addiction Task Force and Prevention leadership group members, and we had a really big meeting, and we talked about the data. We had a lot of data around this stuff. What are we looking at? What stands out? What are the problems? What are the root causes or underlying things, whether they're systems breakdowns or workforce or stigma, things like that. What are the problems, and how do we make changes? What are our strategies? What are some evidence-based strategies?"[102]

And how she did pivot from assessment to action?

"First of all, we assessed each problem and whether we were ready to address the problem," she said. "We might be ready, but is our whole community ready in terms of professional development, community education, outreach, and education, etc.? And then we walked through these planning processes to identify tangible goals and changes that we can make based on the data that we've been given. We're always learning, gleaning, and changing. And repurposing, because we don't have the time to reinvent things. We want to do it for our community, and we want to make it fit in our community."

Identify Potential Coalition Members

Development of the coalition membership, especially in the early stages of the coalition lifecycle when needs are prioritized and strategic goals are being discussed, is a critical exercise that warrants thoughtful consideration. Who are the potential members? What organizations are to be represented? What skills do we seek? How do we conduct outreach and recruit members?

Membership for the coalition should reflect the community the coalition serves. This includes municipal representatives, and sectors such as health, education, workforce, law enforcement, first responders, justice systems, business, and housing. People with lived experience should also be sought out for membership, as they can speak to and represent the realities of substance use as individuals, members of families, and employees. Equally important, members of families impacted by SUD should also be sought out for the coalition. Note that not every member needs to be recruited all at once, nor at the beginning of the formation of the coalition.

Diversity should also reflect the demographics of the community. For the Greater Portsmouth Youth Wellness Coalition, for example, we were told by youth members,

"Nothing about us without us." The message was clear. Membership that included people with lived experience and from underrepresented populations was mandatory.

It is productive to create a summary of the coalition, or what is often referred to as the "elevator pitch," which is nothing more than a summary of the challenge that the coalition strives to address. You should include high-level goals, the skill and talents being sought, the format of the meetings, and the expected time commitments on the part of the membership. This is referred to as an elevator pitch as it is the conversation you'd strike with another person on a one- to two-minute elevator ride.

Coordination and Why It's Important

It is sometimes said that if every community stakeholder is responsible for coordination, then none of the stakeholders are responsible for coordination. Author Alison Jones Webb adds, "When we step back as community members and let treatment providers, social workers, drug court lawyers, judges and health care and other professionals do all the heavy lifting, we shouldn't be surprised when the results fall short. Their collective work, while needed and so beneficial, isn't sufficient to address addiction in our communities.[103]

Community-based research also makes it clear that it is important to invest in creating a collaborative structure that provides facilitation and project management. ORS Impact offers that "creating and managing collective impact requires a separate organization and staff with a very specific set of skills to serve as the backbone for the entire initiative. Coordination takes time, and none of the participating organizations has any to spare. The expectation that collaboration can occur without a supporting infrastructure is one of the most frequent reasons why it fails."[104]

Greater Portsmouth Recovery Coalition leader and Pinetree Institute associate director Molly Louison-Semrow adds, "I know, through a lot of personal experience, that without dedicated, neutral independent facilitation, the coalition is difficult to coordinate. So one of the great things about convening this group is that we at Pinetree have no financial stake in the game, we're not competing for these direct service grants, we're not in any sort of competition with our partners. They're really just our partners. And our role is to promote them and to support them however we can. And these are people doing incredibly, incredibly hard jobs that are really busy, that have tons of clients or that have tons of businesses they are working with. Whatever it may be, we're there solely with the purpose to do this coordination work to bring them together to make sure people are talking to each other and sharing resources. That shouldn't be any one provider's job. It should be an independent job. And I think that's how dedicated facilitation makes it work."[105]

Funding for Coordination

Securing adequate funds is perhaps the most difficult step in building an effective and sustainable coalition. The Greater Portsmouth Recovery Coalition was fortunate to have funding for five years of coordination support from a variety of sources including the City of Portsmouth, Foundation for Seacoast Health, New Hampshire Charitable Foundation, Rotary District 7780, Granite Pathways/Safe Harbor Recovery Center, and an anonymous donor.

Author and professor David Best adds, "The coalition approach suggests a coming together of diverse groups—people in recovery, people who feel they have completed their recovery journeys, family members, professionals, policy makers, and researchers—as well as community activists whose area of interest are unrelated to substance use . . . The challenge, however, is always sustainability and the links this has to issues of resourcing and funding."[106]

Funding from grants, donors, and other foundational benefactors cannot be expected or sustained in perpetuity. At some point after the coalition has resulted in a sufficient level of recovery capacity, that community (town, city, county, state) needs to step up to prioritize the efforts of the coalition as a public safety/public health line item in their respective budgets.

Orient Members to SUD and Evidence-Based Practices

As the coalition grows from the initial steering committee to a broader and deeper group of members, it is time for the coalition to come to a common understanding of the SUD crisis in the community. Perhaps there is a representative organization with deep knowledge of the subject that would be willing to make a presentation to the larger group. Holding a focus group of various SUD-related stakeholders to articulate the challenge in local terms would be effective.

Wherever possible, evidence-based sources should be consulted. SAMHSA, NIDA (the National Institute of Drug Abuse), and NIH (the National Institutes of Health) are reliable sources. To bring it locally, state-level DHHS (Department of Health and Human Services) can be useful. A city or town's publicly available public health reports can often put a spotlight on the local impact of addiction.

Training can provide an influx of new ideas and best practices but does not necessarily need to be in the form of formal presentation of content. Dialogue and conversations can raise the knowledge base of the coalition. Attending conferences and workshops on the part of members is also an effective way to bring new learning into the coalition and to expand the network of subject matter experts.

The coalition can and should be a growth opportunity for members. Skill building can improve the coalition's impact and enhance member retention. For the Greater Portsmouth Recovery Coalition, we used a combination of training programs including all of the above. We also invited licensed professionals to present the science of addiction and effective recovery and treatment options. Over time, the subjects expanded to other related topics such as medication-assisted treatment, harm reduction, and recovery housing.

Develop Coalition Rules of Engagement

How does the coalition work together as a unit? What are the expectations? When do we meet? What is the agenda for upcoming meetings?

Effective community coalitions operate under a common mission and vision. Getting coalition members on the same page is fairly straightforward at the initial convening of the coalition. Having a signed document, at least for members of the coalition's steering committee, helps to ensure that the mission and vision will be adhered to throughout the life of the coalitions. It also provides clarity regarding roles and responsibilities.

Memorandum of Understanding

The Coalition is responsible for:

5. Creating and following bylaws and policies.
6. Formulating coalition goals and objectives.
7. Overseeing operation of activities, programs, and paid staff.
8. Increasing new membership of the coalition.
9. Creating and following a strategic twelve-month action plan.
10. Creating a credible and relevant sustainability plan including volunteer membership and resources, both financial and material.
11. Respecting the rights of coalition members to hold their own opinions and beliefs.
12. Other responsibilities as needed.

NAME, representing SECTOR, is responsible for:

1. Being a community leader among the represented sector.
2. Ensuring clear communication between the sector represented and the coalition.

3. Acting as a positive role model for youth, families, and peers.

4. Supporting the coalition's mission.

5. Attending coalition meetings that are held on a monthly basis.

6. Participating on at least one committee.

7. Attending coalition-sponsored trainings, town hall meetings, and other community events.

8. Contributing to the strategic action planning process.

9. Participating in sustaining the coalition's capacity, involvement, and goals.

10. Using his/her activities as in-kind match, if applicable.

11. Other responsibilities as needed.

Documents and Record Keeping

The coalition should document all official business of the coalition including meeting agendas, minutes, presentations, white papers, etc. All documents should be identified by version, date, and author. Store all documents electronically in a secure location with a backup to the cloud (Dropbox, Google Drive, OneDrive, etc.).

CHAPTER 9

WHY IMPLEMENTING A COMMUNITY COALITION CAN BE SO DIFFICULT

If forming a coalition to address the impact of SUD was a simple exercise, coalitions would exist in nearly every community. After all, most communities have been impacted by addiction. And the motivation is certainly there considering the cost of addiction in terms of lives lost, families destroyed, and the adverse impact to public health, safety, and the local economy.

For more than five years, I've either led or participated in numerous community coalitions. Some have flourished. Others have floundered. Some have had fast starts and lost steam. Still others have started off slowly, only to build momentum over time. Some of the key learnings include a common pattern of barriers to getting a recovery-oriented system of care in motion. These barriers include *stigma*, a *lack of common understanding of the problem*, *where to begin*, *denial* that there is a SUD problem in the first place (I swear this was true in one Seacoast New Hampshire community), the *lack of funding*, and the *lack of coordination*. For some coalitions that did get off the ground, they were not sustained due to *lack of ongoing financial support* over multiple years. Others have floundered because of the *lack of decision makers* participating in the coalition.

The University of Kansas has defined common barriers to coalition building including organizations competing for turf, the history and integrity of the organizations being considered for coalition membership, too many "elites" with impressive degrees that lack lived experience, poor community communication links, lack of capacity, lack of funding, and lack of leadership.[107]

Stigma and the Lack of Common Understanding

"Addiction is a moral failing."

"Throw them all in jail."

"We can't hire a person in recovery as they will congregate in the parking lot and use drugs."

"If we let them build a sober home in our neighborhood, they will soon be selling drugs to our kids."

"Allowing them to put a recovery center in town will only increase drug use in our community."

I have personally heard each of these statements at informational sessions in advance of standing up recovery assets in various communities. I've learned that meeting these people where they are at—listening to their objections, trying to understand what is behind these beliefs, resisting the urge to respond emotionally—is often the only way to gradually open minds. But it can be done.

Merriam-Webster defines "stigma" as a set of negative and unfair beliefs that a society or group of people have about something; a mark of shame or discredit.[108] Taken a step further, stigma can be a major barrier facing individuals and families seeking help for themselves or a loved one dealing with a substance use disorder. The fear of being marginalized, to be seen as a moral failure, or even more nefariously, to be denied basic needs such as employment, housing, and other essential services prevents many from coming forward.

Stigma feeds the common tropes that marginalize the "addict" and the addiction. We live in a society where certain populations of recovering addicts are celebrated as courageous, while others are vilified and judged as a burden on society. Author Leslie Jamison in her remarkable memoir *The Recovering: Intoxication and Its Aftermath*, states it more bluntly: ". . . some addicts get pitied, others get blamed—that it keeps overlapping and evolving to suit our purposes. Alcoholics are tortured geniuses. Drug addicts are deviant zombies. Male drunks are thrilling. Female drunks are bad moms. White addicts get their suffering witnessed. Addicts of color get punished. Celebrity addicts get posh rehab with equine therapy. Poor addicts get hard time."[109]

Contemporary understanding of the impact of substance use disorder has been largely driven by the fact that nearly all of us have our own personal lived experience, a family member, or a friend who has been impacted by addiction. Many of us have been indoctrinated on elements of the recovery continuum of care. Some of us are familiar with recovery housing, medication-assisted treatment, harm reduction, or another provider/community-based organization.

That said, not all of us in the public sphere have the same opinions on what constitutes recovery. Twelve-step programs such as Alcoholics Anonymous are based on abstinence. Others such as SMART Recovery or All Recovery take a more open approach where relapses or setbacks are accepted as the normal course of recovery. A limited focus on abstinence has led to conflict with advocates of 12-step programs when evidence shows that highly effective treatments such as methadone, buprenorphine, and harm reduction have become increasingly accepted in the recovery space.

Another, less nefarious resistance to evidence-based approaches to SUD treatment and recovery is simply a lack of understanding of this evidence. This naivete leads to false beliefs that are perpetuated through our daily conversations and, perhaps more tragically, through social media. As a result, we see common, oft-repeated myths that increase the capacity for stigma, and lead to individuals and families being denied timely and effective care.

In 2019, a substantial group of cross-sector providers, educators, law-enforcement leaders, and municipal workers gathered for what evolved to be known as the Kennebunk (Maine) Coordinated Response to SUD. One of the primary needs identified by that coalition was to provide community education and outreach to address misconceptions, misunderstanding, or sadly, ignorance. A subcommittee was formed to define and counter stigma and misunderstanding. Here is a sampling of those misconceptions:

Common myths:

1. Addiction is not a disease but a moral failing.
2. Recovery homes bring crime into the neighborhood.
3. Medication-Assisted Treatment (MAT) is replacing one drug with another.
4. Harm reduction enables those who use substances.
5. People in recovery are lousy employees.
6. My company does not have a problem with drugs and alcohol.
7. People need to hit rock bottom to get help.
8. Addiction affects only those who use substances.
9. Treatment and recovery are one-size-fits-all.
10. Abstinence is the only acceptable outcome in recovery.
11. We don't have many OD deaths in Kennebunk; therefore, we do not have a problem.

Using these examples as a basis for raising the community's understanding of the realities of addiction in the community can go a long way to eliminating opposition to community coalitions.

Where to Begin

From my experience, convening a small but representative group of leaders and influencers is the easiest way to get the ball rolling. We've covered the best practices for building a coalition, but putting these approaches into real-life situations can sometimes be daunting. What to do when you get the right people together can set the tone (positive or otherwise) for early convenings. The following example of the Lewiston-Auburn Area Recovery Collaborative demonstrates an effective approach for starting a coalition to address substance use.

Case Study: Lewiston-Auburn Area Recovery Collaborative

Healthy Androscoggin is a nonprofit agency in Lewiston, Maine, which provides accessible healthy living services to Androscoggin County in south-central Maine. Auburn is its county seat, and its largest city is Lewiston. The Lewiston-Auburn community refers to the greater metropolitan area of the two cities. Many of the health-related social services and community-based organizations support and serve both cities. Healthy Androscoggin "works to ensure that Androscoggin County residents have equitable access to the resources they need to lead healthy lives."[110]

The L-A community is perhaps one of the most diverse communities in the northeast on a per-capita basis. The community intentionally conducts outreach for and welcomes so-called "new Mainers" from across the globe. These immigrants arrive from Ukraine, Afghanistan, Somalia, Central America, and many other countries, knowing that they will have a safe community that is purposefully providing culturally appropriate services for integration.

Healthy Androscoggin has been awarded a grant to build capacity for addiction prevention, treatment, and recovery for the county, and has formed a robust coalition using principles described in Chapter 8. Their journey to build a coalition is a great example of a Recovery Ready Community in progress.

Rowan McFadden is a Maine Certified Prevention Specialist whose day job is Health Promotion Coordinator at Healthy Androscoggin. McFadden is the facilitator for the Lewiston-Auburn Area Recovery Collaborative and spends about 50 percent of his work capacity leading the coalition.

Jennifer Edwards is the public health manager for the city of Auburn. Edwards said, "I work for Auburn's Business and Community Development Department, which houses general assistance and community development for the city. Part of our job is to oversee community block grants that run through our department."[111]

Sustainability is a real concern for the coalition, which recently completed its Assessment and Planning phases of the program. "The coalition is currently funded through calendar year 2026," McFadden said during my recent visit to Auburn. "We hope to secure additional funding through the state as part of the next round of grants being offered to recovery communities across the state."

Other challenges include sustainable subcommittees, continued commitment for members beyond 2025, and especially the lack of community decision makers at the committee leadership level. "Our current membership is doing a great job with boots-on-the-street activities, but in many cases they don't have the ability to make decisions on behalf of their organization. We are never really certain how much of what gets shared in the meeting trickles up in conversations in a manner that a decision maker is going to feel like they can help with this."

"What would be your strategy to approach decision makers?" I asked.

"We've talked about doing a key stakeholder meeting, to get the right people present and perhaps call it a key stakeholder meeting, or call it an advisory board that gets the decision makers in a room to explain that this is all the stuff that's going on, these are our priorities," McFadden said.

"What are the intended outcomes for the coalition?" I asked.

"That's what we're kind of focusing on right now, especially now that we've finished our Overdose Prevention and Response plan. So really, the big one is, do we see a reduction in fatal and non-fatal overdoses in Androscoggin County once we start to implement our strategic priorities?"

Coalition Representation[112]

Healthy Androscoggin assumed facilitation of the Lewiston-Auburn Area Recovery Coalition (LAARC) following their grant award from Maine's Project to Prevent Prescription Drug/Opioid Overdose-Related Deaths. This funding allowed for more focused efforts within the community coalition to respond to Androscoggin County's high rates of fatal and nonfatal overdoses. The collaborative focused on connecting individuals and organizations interested in furthering the efforts to promote, educate, prevent, and respond to the multifaceted problems associated with substance use across Androscoggin County. The composition of the coalition was:

- City of Auburn

- City of Lewiston

- Maine Re-Entry Network

- Better Life Partners

- *Journey* magazine
- Androscoggin County Vocational Rehabilitation
- Pinetree Institute
- Auburn YMCA
- Generational Noor
- Maine Community Integration
- Church of Safe Injection
- Androscoggin County Jail
- Community Concepts
- Spurwink
- New Beginnings
- Poland High School
- Lewiston High School
- New Ventures Maine
- Lewiston Career Center
- Others

Funding

This program is funded and supported by Maine's Project to Prevent Prescription Drug/Opioid Overdose-Related Deaths.

Objective

To reduce overdose deaths and substance use-related harms over the next three to five years. Note that the objective is SMART: Specific, Measurable, Achievable, Relevant, Time-Bound.

Assessment

- Demographically, Androscoggin County—both for the metropolitan Lewiston-Auburn community and especially rural regions of the county—have been disproportionately impacted by the Maine opioid crisis.

- In 2022, there were 19.7 overdoses per 1000 residents in Androscoggin County. This was the second highest rate of overdose in the state.

- From January to May 2024, there have been 304 nonfatal and 18 fatal overdoses in Androscoggin County. This is representative of 10 percent of the total number of fatal and nonfatal overdoses statewide.

- Additional risks and harms, such as infectious diseases, infants born exposed to substances, and improperly disposed syringe waste are associated with substance use disorder. These risks and harms impact individuals, families, and the Androscoggin community at large.

- In Androscoggin County there have been higher rates of infants born exposed to substances since 2023.

- From 2019 to 2023, 13.7 percent of live births in Androscoggin County were substance exposed births.

- The 2021 Maine Integrated Youth Health Survey showed that students are being offered substances on school grounds at higher rates than any other county in the state of Maine.

- 17.6 percent of high school students and 7 percent of middle school students in Androscoggin County have been offered substances on school grounds in the past twelve months, compared to the state average of 16.9 percent for high schoolers and 5.4 percent for middle schoolers.[113] [114]

Guiding Principles of the Coalition[115]

1. **Advance Health Equity:** Any strategies implemented must seek to increase equitable access to resources needed for positive health outcomes and recognize disproportionately affected populations' unique experiences and needs to develop targeted interventions.

2. **Address Social Determinants of Health:** To address the overdose crisis, it is critical to see the larger context in which the crisis is occurring and seek to mitigate underlying risk factors. We must recognize the role of social determinants of health in prevention and intervention.

3. **Build Community Capacity and Empowerment:** Engaging communities in this work is critical to success. Helping community members understand their role in the solutions that can improve conditions—not just for individuals at risk of overdose, but the whole community—is vital.

4. **Increase Coordination and Collaboration:** Tackling complex issues requires a systemic approach. This necessitates developing infrastructure that builds

on past success and supports meaningful collaboration within Androscoggin County and amongst community partners with a focus on efficiency and cohesion.

5. **Enhance Data-Driven Decision-Making:** Make program, municipal, state, and national data available to drive program change and improvement. Increase the capacity of stakeholders to move from data collection to data analysis to data-guided action.

Strategic Priorities

The focus of the coalition is to build a six-pillar strategic plan. Each of the strategic focus areas includes an identification of gaps, inventory of existing assets or capabilities, and a set of recommendations for going forward. The six pillars are:

1. Education and Engagement
2. Prevention
3. Harm Reduction
4. Treatment
5. Recovery

Below is an example of the strategic planning for *Harm Reduction*:

Strategic Statement

Sustain and expand existing harm reduction efforts, especially in areas experiencing high overdose rates and populations at high risk for negative consequences of drug use. Improve public safety response to overdoses through increased education, stigma reduction, transparency, and acceptance of best practices.

Gaps

- There continues to be barriers for rural community members in accessing harm reduction services, the most significant being transportation accessibility.
- Safe syringe disposal options are limited to the greater Lewiston/Auburn area.
- There are a lack of syringe disposal options in public restrooms and other public places.

- It continues to be a challenge to engage the larger community within Andro-scoggin County in educational opportunities on the basics of harms caused by substances and risks associated with substance use due to the associated stigma.

- Individuals without independent communication technology face significant barriers in accessing communication technology, and thus care.

- Culturally competent harm reduction education for Androscoggin County's diverse demographics is lacking.

- There are barriers to accessing the most up-to-date communication around quantifying overdose fatalities and non-fatalities in Androscoggin County, spe-cifically, regarding additional risks within the drug supply for the greater Andro-scoggin County public.

- There is a lack of overdose data that provides demographic detail, specifically regarding race and other information that would assist in identifying overdose prevalence among our New Mainer communities.

- There are currently very limited options for harm reduction services for youth.

- Limited funding and continued stigma has made it difficult to broaden harm reduction activities, particularly when it comes to safer use supplies such as dis-posable pipes.

Assets and Capabilities

- Church of Safe Injection (CoSI) Safe Syringe Program and Wound Care

- Spurwink Safe Syringe Program and Harm Reduction Program

- Fourteen syringe disposal boxes in Lewiston

- Seventeen Tier 2 Naloxone Distributors in Androscoggin County

- The Drop-In Center located in Auburn hosts community providers on Wednes-day mornings offering a stable and regular connection point for unhoused com-munity members to meet with a variety of community providers. These include OPTIONS (Overdose Prevention Through Intensive Outreach) liaisons, Project Support You workers, and case managers. This program has been very successful and should be expanded.

- CoSI community member and organizational staff trainings, overdose recogni-tion and reversal

- CoSI Peer Navigation Services

- OPTIONS liaisons at Spurwink Services
- *Journey* magazine
- Statewide SPIKE Alert by Text system that alerts individuals to upticks in overdoses
- Project Support You
- OPTIONS for Androscoggin County

Recommendations

- Support the creation of a Mobile Health Unit to address health needs of those who are unable to or have had negative experiences in traditional healthcare settings.
- CoSI harm reduction focused Community Drop-In Center.
- Increase general community education opportunities on the basics of harm reduction and its philosophy.
- Support the creation of low-barrier, secular shelter/treatment beds.
- Locate funding for mobile phones/connectivity technology.
- Provide needle cleanup and syringe cleanup hotlines and identify a lead organization willing to manage the hotline. This would allow community members to call in and request needle and syringe cleanup within Androscoggin County.
- Expansion of SPIKE system to include supply updates.
- Support improved communication mechanisms across systems to ensure data sharing to better inform intervention and prevention strategies utilized throughout Androscoggin County.

Lessons Learned

1. **Representation:** Ensure recruiting sector decision makers for coalition leadership committees.
2. **Sustainability:** Seek multi-year funding sources for the coalition to ensure year-to-year continuity.
3. **Coordination:** Coordination of the coalition is no one's job if it is everyone's job. Ensure there is funding for a neutral-party coordination role.

SECTION 3

THE RECOVERY READY COMMUNITY

CHAPTER 10

WHAT IS A RECOVERY READY COMMUNITY?

Well, it depends.

In my twelve-plus years of experience and taking into account the countless discussions I've had with community coalitions and recovery professionals over that time period, I can speak with confidence that there cannot be a single numerical standard for designating a community as "recovery ready." Yes, there are common elements of what constitutes a so-called Recovery Ready Community, but there are also many variables including community culture, government structure, socioeconomic status, diversity (or lack thereof), geographical location, and many other nuances that define a community's identity.

Recovery readiness to a large extent, is what a community says it is. What works for the city of Portsmouth, a city of twenty-two thousand on the Seacoast in New Hampshire, does not necessarily work for Columbus, Ohio, or Louisville, Kentucky. Recovery readiness is what that community decides for itself in the form of a common vision and measurable outcomes. Recovery readiness is about the journey, not the destination. Communities that are self-aware, that are working on community issues, and that are bringing different stakeholders together to address the impact of addiction in their community may be sufficient for that community's level of readiness.

I offered this argument to Robin Rieske, MS, who is a certified prevention specialist and community consultant based in Brattleboro, Vermont. "Exactly," was Rieske's reply. "And it's all about that level of readiness. Like in some communities, it might just be having information about what recovery is, and for other communities, it's about having low-barrier recovery housing. So, it just depends on the need and your community."[116]

I posed the same point to Dr. Alex Elswick from the University of Kentucky. He responded, "In Kentucky, one of the tensions we had to figure out was you can't have the same standard in Lexington, Kentucky that you do in Pike County. They are completely different communities, and it isn't fair to Pikeville, where they have different resources, different cultures, have different needs, different population, different demographics, they're in a different time and place to your point. Yes, different attitudes towards different interventions and all the way down the line."[117]

"In public health, we see individuals as part of a complex web of individual characteristics, family relationships, social networks, cultural norms, and economic factors that create the social determinants of health," says author Alison Jones Webb in her book *Recovery Allies: How to Support Addiction and Build Recovery-Friendly Communities*.[118] "It is about mobilizing community capital and making it accessible to people who don't have connections or resources to get the support and assistance they need for their recovery."

Just as recovery looks different for different individuals, recovery looks different for each community. Community recovery is meeting the community "where it's at," leveraging the strengths, as individuals self-define the meaning of recovery in their terms, communities can define recovery on their terms as well.

It is important to note, however, that this self-determining approach to defining a recovery-ready community does not eliminate the need to define a minimum and common components of a recovery ready community. Nor does it ignore the need for the coalition to define and measure outcomes at the outset and measure along the journey to becoming recovery-ready.

Commonly Well CEO David Whitesock weighed in on the importance of defining and measuring outcomes. "I think each community is going to be a little bit different. If you sit down with community A and community B, community A might say, 'The thing that we really got to focus on is employment.' Community B is going to say 'No, it's transportation. People can't get from A to B. Everybody's got a job. They just can't get there.' Those outcomes matter because that becomes the key factor that drives all the other actions."[119]

I also posed the question about the measurement of recovery readiness to Aaron Williams, senior advisor at the National Council for Mental Wellbeing, and co-author of the Trauma Informed Recovery Oriented System of Care (TI-ROSC) Toolkit. "I think that's a good way to think about it. We worked on a paper for the Peer Recovery Center of Excellence about this idea of recovery readiness and recovery consciousness. The TI-ROSC program is designed to provide general knowledge on trauma and substance use, to help communities think through that and understand better, where the field is, what's the current state, what's happening in their own communities. We take that information and then we tailor the program to those communities."[120]

On the importance of adapting to the needs of the community, Lisa Attygalle of Tamarack Institute said, "One of the principles for our work is that place really matters. We can't just replicate what works for one community to work for all communities. We can replicate a lot of an approach, but you can't replicate all of an approach, because place is really important. The assets are different. What the community cares about is different. Some communities are more risk tolerant than others. The culture is different."[121]

Recovery "Ready" or Recovery "Friendly"?

What is the difference between the terms Recovery *Friendly* Community versus Recovery *Ready* Community? The national Recovery Ready Workplace (RRW) initiative, which is largely based on the pioneering work of New Hampshire's Recovery Friendly Workplace (RFW), equates the two versions, and grandfathers state designation for existing Recovery Friendly Workplaces within their respective states.[122]

That said, I believe there is nuanced difference between the word *friendly* versus the word *ready* that is worth discussing. *Friendly* denotes something that is "not causing or likely to cause harm." For example, "an eco-*friendly* vehicle."[123] Conversely, the word *ready* refers to an entity being "prepared for immediate use" or "immediately available," as in "dinner is *ready*" or "had *ready* cash."[124]

For the purpose of this book, Recovery Ready Communities have resources and capacity and are mobilized for action. Recovery Friendly Communities are communities that have not yet taken the steps necessary to build that capacity. Therefore, this book is a practical guide to building Recovery *Ready* Communities.

Recovery Consciousness

The concept of recovery consciousness helps to zoom in on the fundamental requirements of a recovery ready community, building on the value and power of people with lived experience who live there. In the Peer Recovery Center of Excellence report *Increasing Recovery Consciousness: Grounding Systems in Recovery*, the importance of people with lived experience in recovery systems is made clear: "Implicit within the peer model is a different way of working with and relating to individuals and communities. It is about centering the lived experiences of addiction and recovery, or lived experiences of mental health challenges and recovery, and using those lenses to see and reframe everything that a program, organization, institution, or system does. When we understand that, it becomes easier to discern which programs are truly offering recovery support services (RSS) and others that aspire to deliver RSS but have changed their practices to be consistent with the principles of recovery. True recovery support isn't just about what organizations do; it is about how they do it."[125]

Recovery consciousness within a system of care is greater than the sum of its parts. We have seen communities come together to marshal resources towards specific crises such as overdoses, homelessness, recovery in the workforce, transmission of infectious disease, etc. There are certainly elements of recovery consciousness within these discrete efforts. However, where is the coordination between these efforts? Where are people with lived experience, or better yet where are people who *are still using drugs* involved in the system of care to provide context and to inform?

To answer these questions, we again refer to the Peer Recovery Center of Excellence report: "First and foremost, the work (of the recovery-oriented system of care) is centered in the lived and living experience of persons in recovery. This means that all aspects of the organization—its mission, vision, culture, infrastructure, policies and practices, governance, leadership, and staffing—are infused with the core philosophies and values that use lived/living experience perspectives to ground all aspect of the organization and its work."[126]

There can be no recovery ready community without recovery consciousness.

CHAPTER 11

THE RECOVERY READY COMMUNITY MODEL

What is a Recovery-Oriented System of Care?

One of the long-lasting messages I heard during my two-month stint in rehab was that on average it could take up to two years for my brain to heal from my opioid addiction, and up to five years to achieve successful long-term recovery. I freaked. I wanted it to heal now. Stat!

Looking back on my own journey of long-term recovery, I now understand that I could not have achieved that accomplishment without the support of my family and my recovery community, especially during those first five years. By "my recovery community," I refer to my place of employment, physical and mental health providers, peer recovery supports, and mutual assistance organizations such as Alcoholics Anonymous, Al-Anon, Narcotics Anonymous, and Heroin Anonymous. This list of community supports from which I benefitted is noteworthy because these were the only resources that were available to me in 2012 when I got sober.

I was fortunate in that I had a home and my family to return to, my job waiting for me, and health insurance that enabled me to continue my treatment and recovery protocols following my out-of-state inpatient treatment. Had I needed a bed at a recovery home, interventions such as harm reduction, and/or medication-assisted treatment, I would have been out of luck. Had I been found to have had drug paraphernalia on my person, I probably would have been arrested and publicly humiliated by having my name and picture in the paper. Had I overdosed, I would have likely died since overdose reversal drugs such as Narcan were not yet available. Recalling those early days, it is quite likely that I would have slipped through the cracks of traditional care and become another statistic. My family would have been stigmatized. Perhaps they would have been shunned due to the lack of understanding of addiction being a diagnosable chronic illness.

Statistically, the successful recovery of individuals with SUD is positively impacted by the use of medical, community, and social supports, especially within the first five years of the recovery process. Further, as Ashford et al. suggest, "long-term supports will be the most beneficial when they exist within an individual's local community."[127]

The challenge is to find an approach that assists communities to identify recovery assets, and that develops a process for identifying gaps, barriers, and other unmet needs for individuals and their families to get the help they need.

In a 2010 resource guide, SAMHSA defines a *Recovery-Oriented System of Care (ROSC)* as a "coordinated network of community-based services and supports that is person-centered and builds on the strengths and resiliencies of individuals, families, and communities to achieve abstinence and improved health, wellness, and quality of life for those with or at risk of alcohol and drug problems."[128] In this example, the continuum of care for recovery-oriented activities can be divided into four categories: Prevention, Intervention, Treatment, and Post-Treatment.

The United States surgeon general, in his 2016 report *Facing Addiction in America: The Surgeon General's Report on Alcohol, Drugs, and Health*, defines a "continuum of care" as an integrated system of care that guides and tracks a person over time through a comprehensive array of health services appropriate to the individual's need, and that may include prevention, early intervention, treatment, continuing care and recovery support.[129] Applying this definition to the SUD continuum of care, the report specifies the following five elements of the continuum:

1. Enhancing Health

2. Primary Prevention

3. Early Intervention

4. Treatment

5. Recovery Support

Author David Best, from his book *Pathways to Recovery and Desistance*, "the key ideas here (recovery-oriented systems of care) are partnerships: consultant relationships, systems anchored in the community, integrated services, inclusion of the voices of recovery individuals and their families, and strengths-based working."[130]

It should be apparent that there are multiple approaches to building a recovery-oriented system of care. Before I apply these principles to a common set of elements for a Recovery Ready Community, let's first consider a trauma-informed approach.

Trauma-Informed Recovery Oriented Systems of Care

The pervasiveness of trauma of varying degrees and types within our communities, as well as the importance of organizations to realize, recognize, respond, and resist re-traumatization is well established. The principles of trauma-informed care help organizations to reflect on an overarching framework or "lens" through which policies/procedures/processes, behaviors and interactions are filtered.[131]

Taking the Recovery-Oriented System of Care to another level, the National Council for Mental Wellbeing is a nonprofit membership organization that drives policy and social change on behalf of more than thirty-four hundred mental health and substance use treatment organizations across the United States. The organization offers consulting services with a focus on public policy, workforce development, public health, equity, and integrated health.

One of the notable programs of the organization is the 2022 publication of the Trauma-Informed Recovery-Oriented System of Care Toolkit.[132] The toolkit was developed in collaboration with the state of Indiana with eighteen (of ninety-nine) counties receiving training and technical assistance from the organization.

The toolkit uses the SAMHSA definition of a *trauma-informed approach* as "a program, organization or system that recognizes the widespread impact of trauma and understands potential paths for recovery; recognizes the signs and symptoms of trauma in clients, families, staff and others involved with the system; and responds by fully integrating knowledge about trauma into policies, procedures and practices and seeks to actively resist re-traumatization."[133]

Example: Dearborn County (Indiana)

The Community Action Recovery Effort (CARE) of Dearborn County is a wonderful example of a Recovery Oriented System of Care and is comprised of diverse stakeholders coming together to support community wellness and ensure a recovery ready community. Their mission statement is county-centric: "Dearborn is an educated and unified community where individuals and families can safely and easily access reliable services and lasting support towards hope, recovery and meaning in life."[134] The Dearborn County CARE has implemented a social media and digital marketing approach including webinars and an interactive website to connect county residents to trauma-informed services and support. Their website provides a link for local services and support with contact information for each.

The CARE program is also comprised of work groups that address specific areas within the continuum of care. Each of these work groups have goal statements, list successes, and identify future plans.

CARE Work Groups

- **Stigma and Awareness:** Increase awareness and understanding of addiction science, recovery, services available and the benefits of evidence-based treatments through a stigma busting campaign.

- **Screening:** Ensure all Dearborn County residents who are at risk are screened for trauma and substance use disorders at schools, primary care, clinics, and hospitals.

- **Recovery Hub:** Establish a Recovery Hub to house ROSC services and supports.

- **Transportation Work Group:** Ensure all Dearborn County residents have access to low-cost/no-cost transportation to access their medical appointments, and maintenance and sustainability recovery supports.

- **Peer Recovery Supports:** Ensure Dearborn County residents have access to necessary peer recovery supports for recovery and reconnection.

- **Recovery Housing:** Ensure Dearborn County residents in recovery have access to housing.

What follows is a proposed model for a Recovery Ready Community using the Trauma-Informed Recovery-Oriented Systems of Care (TI-ROSC) as a basis for understanding the recovery continuum of care, and the corresponding recovery assets of a community using the experiences of multiple community coalitions such as the Greater Portsmouth Recovery Coalition and the Lewiston-Auburn Area Recovery Collaborative.

Common Elements of Recovery Ready Community
Portsmouth, New Hampshire

Although there are a myriad of systems-level approaches for implementing Recovery-Oriented Systems of Care, there are common elements that can be adapted to fit the needs of a given community. For the coalitions that Pinetree Institute has coordinated and continues to lead in New Hampshire and Maine, we've found that Recovery Ready Communities provide coordinated community-based services that are person-centered and build strength and resilience of individuals, families, and communities. What we've found is that a recovery ready framework needs to address the entire continuum of care of *prevention*, *harm reduction*, *treatment*, and *recovery support*, including re-entry into the community.

The figure below illustrates the Greater Portsmouth Recovery Coalition model for a recovery continuum of care. I will use the Greater Portsmouth Recovery Coalition model as the basis for the case study.

At Pinetree Institute, we coordinated the Greater Portsmouth Recovery Community, a coalition that was founded in 2019, where we field tested a model for a Recovery Ready Community to serve *individuals*, *families*, and *affected others*.[135] This model was developed

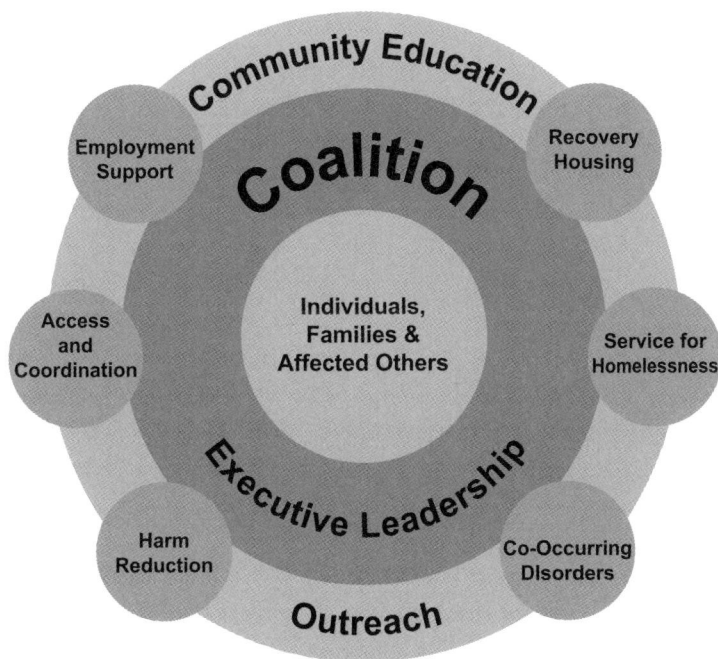

Figure 2: Greater Portsmouth Recovery Coalition Framework
(copyright Pinetree Institute, 2024).

and adapted over time to meet the needs of the greater Seacoast community of New Hampshire. Through initial assessment and evaluation of these stated needs the coalition finalized the basic elements of a Recovery Ready Community: *recovery housing, access to and coordination of services, employment support, harm reduction, services for the homeless,* and *services for co-occurring disorders.* Other communities may and will likely have other priority focus areas. Finally, the surrounding circle emphasizes the need for *community education* to address stigma, and *outreach* programs to inform the community of the important work of the coalition.

York County, Maine

In 2020, Pinetree Institute also facilitated an assessment of needs in southern Maine with the communities of Kennebunk, Kennebunkport, and Arundel. The Kennebunk Coordinated Response to SUD was established with local and regional stakeholders that served the greater Kennebunk community. Several priorities emerged from the needs assessment: *recovery housing, employment, transportation, community education,* and *coordination of services.*

Kennebunk is located in York County, which is the southernmost county in Maine. Work is currently underway at Pinetree, funded by the state's attorney general's office, to lead a county-wide assessment of needs to address SUD. Concurrent with this effort is the construction of a forty-five-million-dollar treatment and recovery center adjacent to the York County Corrections facility. The center will provide short- and long-term residential treatment, withdrawal management, recovery housing, and recovery services to former county jail inmates as they continue their treatment and recovery journeys. The complex will also provide the same services for those in need from the general public.[136] Although the assessment phase of the coalition is in its infancy, the coalition is focusing on specific assets, capabilities and gaps around *prevention*, *housing*, *workforce development*, *harm reduction*, *justice systems*, *recovery support* and *treatment system*. In other words, following the same trauma-informed recovery system of care.

State of Maine

Gordon Smith, Maine's director of opioid response, is responsible for coordinating and directing Maine's response to the opioid crisis, including prescriber education and reduction of opioid prescribing, prevention and treatment of substance use disorder, and harm reduction strategies. Gordon was appointed to this role in February 2019 when Governor Janet Mills issued Executive Order 2: An Order to Implement Immediate Responses to Maine's Opioid Epidemic.[137]

Under Smith's leadership, the administration has developed an Opioid Response Strategic Plan that has been updated in 2021 to address challenges stemming from the COVID-19 pandemic and the increased prevalence of lethal non-pharmaceuticals such as fentanyl.[138]

I met with Director Smith in his office in August 2024 to ask for his views on the minimum requirements of a recovery ready community.

He said, "(Recovery communities) start from different places, but you'd still want to see the same elements. *Housing*. *Employment*. I'd want to see *treatment resources*. I'd want to see *recovery community centers* that are welcoming, that are not necessarily treatment centers. I'd want to see a lot of community activities that are addressing *stigma*. For treatment facilities, I'd want to see access to *detox*, and to the full continuum of services, from medically supervised *withdrawal management* to short-term residential to long-term *residential inpatient treatment*, to outpatient facilities, and long-term *recovery support*, and then community support for people in their recovery, *recovery coaches*, certainly want to see *recovery residences*. Now I say access to them doesn't need to mean that they necessarily are going to be located in that community, but you'd want to see these facilities promoted so that people had access to them, and they wouldn't be too far away."

He continued: "I'd want to see a welcoming *governing body of the town*, whether it's selectpersons or whether it's a city council, so that there's not a lot of nimbyism. I'd want to see access to buprenorphine and methadone. So that's *harm reduction*. I'd like to see a *syringe program.* And I'd also want to see a robust array of *prevention* activities, both primary and secondary, after school, before school, in school, and all those community youth development organizations, YMCA, boys clubs, girls 4H and all those mentoring, youth mentoring organizations."[139]

Leslie Clark is executive director of Portland Recovery Community Center (PRCC) in Portland, Maine. PRCC is contracted by the State of Maine to oversee a so-called Recovery Hub of twenty-one recovery community organizations across the Pine Tree state. When I shared with her my conversation with Gordon Smith about defining the minimum requirements of a recovery ready community, we had an in-depth conversation about access to services, and specifically about *navigation* of those services.

"I don't think we talk enough about access and the role of the recovery community organization to help people access services. Within an RCO, people are coming in, family members calling, and we help them connect to those resources. The RCO is really the hub of recovery within that community. It's where all of these elements within the recovery ready community converge. The RCO is there for the individual and their family to find the appropriate community resources throughout their entire journey."[140]

"The *recovery navigator* is someone who is community-based who understands all of the area resources and can direct individuals and families to the network of coordinated services so that people can access what they need: treatment, harm reduction, recovery, support services, housing, transportation, all those kinds of things."

We can now define the minimum elements of a recovery ready community.

Minimum Elements of a Recovery Ready Community

Based on several coalitions I've personally been a part of and based on numerous interviews I've conducted with leaders involved with building recovery capacity within their community or state, the following have emerged as the *minimum elements of a recovery ready community*. Some communities have different programming or services under these categories or have different names. However, the essence of these other community approaches align with the model. It is worth noting that community programs and services need to be adapted to and inclusive of all populations within the community, utilizing culturally appropriate methods.

Minimal Elements of a Recovery Ready Community:

1. Youth Programming
2. Harm Reduction

3. Community Education & Outreach

4. Medication-Assisted Treatment (MAT)

5. In-Patient Treatment

6. Out-patient Treatment

7. Treatment Courts

8. Recovery Housing

9. Recovery Community Organizations

10. Recovery Employment

11. Access to Services

12. Re-Entry Services

13. Peer Recovery Coaches

14. Recovery Community Navigator

These elements would align with the Recovery-Oriented System of Care as illustrated below:

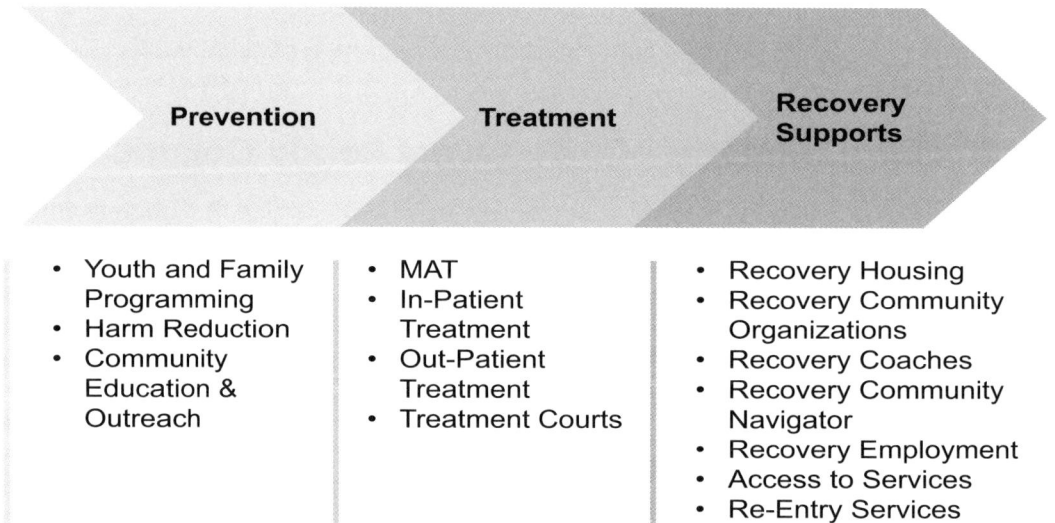

Prevention	Treatment	Recovery Supports
• Youth and Family Programming • Harm Reduction • Community Education & Outreach	• MAT • In-Patient Treatment • Out-Patient Treatment • Treatment Courts	• Recovery Housing • Recovery Community Organizations • Recovery Coaches • Recovery Community Navigator • Recovery Employment • Access to Services • Re-Entry Services

Figure 3: Recovery Ready Community Continuum of Care.

CHAPTER 12

BREAKING IT DOWN

A cursory search for "recovery continuum of care models" will yield a number of frameworks that define the flow (usually left to right) of services, community-based organizations, and other interventions for individuals and families seeking help for addiction-related issues. The challenge of many of these models is that they imply a production line approach to recovery. They don't, however, convey the important message that there are multiple pathways to recovery, and taken further, there are many doorways into the system of care. And since some in recovery experience a recurrence of their drug use, entry points into the system will likely vary for many individuals. It is worthwhile, therefore, to illustrate again the Greater Portsmouth Recovery Coalition model that is adapted from Recovery Ready Continuum of Care model in figure 1. With this approach for a recovery ready community coalition, it is implicit that one can enter into this system of care at any entry point in the continuum of care. It is also clear that there is no finish line. Refer back to figure 1.

SAMHSA's Strategic Prevention Framework[141]

Most of the coalitions I've been involved with have adopted all or a subset of the SAM-HSA Strategic Prevention Framework, a blueprint developed by SAMHSA. Some of these coalitions have done so intentionally and others unintentionally. The Strategic Prevention Framework is based on five sequential steps:

1. **Assessment:** Identify local needs based on data. Assess risk and protective factors.

2. **Capacity:** Build local resources and readiness to address community needs.

3. **Planning:** Find out what works to address prevention needs and how to do it well.

4. **Implementation:** Deliver evidence-based programs and practices as intended.

5. **Evaluation:** Examine the process and outcomes of programs and practices.

Interwoven are two principles that are integrated across each of the steps of the framework:

1. **Cultural competence:** the ability of an individual or organization to understand and interact effectively with people who have different values, lifestyles, and traditions based on their distinctive heritage and social relationships.

2. **Sustainability:** the process of building an adaptive and effective system that achieves and maintains desired long-term results.

Phase 1: Assessment

Assessment is the discovery phase. What is the urgent problem or opportunity to be addressed? What are the needs, barriers, and gaps preventing the community from addressing the problem or pursuing the opportunity? What are the desired outcomes?

Effective assessments should be local to the coalition's catchment area but could be compared with other state or national populations that follow the same criteria. The purpose of the assessment is to gain an understanding of the issues that the coalition will address and provide contextual data for analyzing patterns and setting priorities for prevention programs.

Example: Greater Portsmouth Youth Wellness Coalition: Getting to 'Y'

The Greater Portsmouth Youth Wellness Coalition (GPYWC) is an example of a community coming together to connect children and adolescents with programs within Seacoast New Hampshire communities. The coalition is a partnership of youth, residents, schools, community organizations, businesses, and other partners who are invested in the future of the Greater Portsmouth area. The coalition provides ways for the community to share information and access resources, while supporting initiatives to strengthen the health, well-being, and success of children, youth, and their families. The Greater Portsmouth Youth Wellness Coalition uses the SAMHSA Strategic Prevention Framework as the foundation for its efforts.

One of the lessons learned from the GPYWC is that youth in the community want to be heard. With youth in mind, the Greater Portsmouth Youth Wellness Coalition has included students as members not only of the coalition writ large, but also have a seat on the Steering Committee.

Getting to 'Y' is a national program whereby youth bring meaning to their Youth Risk Behavior Survey data; it is offered by UP for Learning, a Vermont nonprofit organization that assists schools across the United States to engage youth in their own learning.[142] In early 2024, the Greater Portsmouth Youth Wellness Coalition held a Getting to 'Y' retreat with local high school students, during which the group looked at 2021 YRBS data from their school, identified strengths and concerns, and brainstormed root causes.

Phase 2: Capacity

Capacity is where we begin to strengthen existing services and build new resources to achieve the outcomes defined in the assessment phase. How ready is the coalition to pursue the opportunity or address the urgent problem at hand? Is the community aware of the issue or opportunity?

In Chapter 7 we introduced recovery capital. Applying recovery capital to the SAMHSA Strategic Prevention Framework, it follows that capacity involves engaging with community stakeholders, developing and strengthening a prevention team, and raising community awareness. In the SUD prevention realm, capacity specifically refers to those assets and resources that strengthen the ability of a community to prevent downstream mental health and substance use in the first place. The scientific evidence tells us that the most effective programs and resources to prevent substance use mitigate the impact of childhood trauma in the home and in the community.

Earlier in this book we discussed the importance of positive experiences and programming as protective factors to offset the impact of adverse childhood experiences, which in turn reduces health and behavioral issues as our children grow. Any discussion about building capacity to prevent substance use among our young population begins with interdicting adverse childhood experiences. Parental buffering against adverse childhood experiences with the support of community programming has been proven to offset high school drop-out rates, alcohol and drug use, criminal behavior, and mental health challenges.[143] These factors create an environment of safety and belonging to the world outside the four walls of the home:

- **Emotional Support:** feeling social/emotional support and hope.
- **Multiple Sources of Help:** two or more people who give concrete help when needed.
- **Reciprocity:** watching out for each other and doing favors for one another.
- **Social Bridging:** reaching outside the social circle to get help for family or friends.

According to the Search Institute, a nonprofit organization with more than sixty years of research promoting positive youth development, "Developmental Relationships are the roots of thriving and resilience for young people, regardless of their background or circumstances. Through these relationships, young people discover who they are, cultivate abilities to shape their own lives, and learn how to engage with and contribute to the world around them."[144]

Characteristics of developmental relationships:

- **Express Care:** Show me that I matter to you.
- **Challenge Growth:** Push me to keep getting better.
- **Provide Support:** Help me complete tasks and achieve goals.
- **Share Power:** Treat me with respect and give me a say.
- **Expand Possibilities:** Connect me with people and places that broaden my world.

As an example of what these developmental relationships might look like in practice, in my book *A Place in Time: Youth, Community & Baseball,* I wrote about my reflections as a fifteen-year old returning to my hometown after winning the Massachusetts State Babe Ruth Baseball championship:

> *As a representative of our town all-star team, I learned about honor. My actions both in and out of uniform reflected on the city of Leominster, our league, my parents, and my teammates. Our community cared deeply about our successes. They held banquets and lavished awards and ceremonies to recognize our achievement.*
>
> *Looking back with pride on our accomplishments and how they affected the community that rallied behind us, I can appreciate the factors that allowed me to be part of this special experience. Hence the lesson of gratitude for those who supported us along the way: the parents, the neighbors, the businesses, volunteers, and officials that shared in the glory of that place in time.*[145]

Prevention resources and assets that build civic pride and connection to the community can check all the boxes for creating prevention capacity for our kids. However, without a coordinated approach within the community, at-risk youth who fall through the cracks of the system may face health and social challenges as they grow older.

According to the National Council for Mental Wellbeing's Center of Excellence for Integrated Health Solutions, "youth with SUDs experience higher rates of physical and psychiatric illnesses, which diminish overall health and wellbeing. Major depression and anxiety disorders typically emerge during adolescence and can be exacerbated by SUDs, leading to self-injury, academic failure, violence, and suicide. . . . These health consequences underscore the critical need for targeted intervention and support to mitigate these health disparities."[146]

A community coalition approach to intervention that takes into account childhood trauma and provides that community's youth with developmental programming during their formative years, will have a profound impact on negative outcomes for their kids. The Greater Portsmouth Youth Wellness Coalition is a great example of building prevention capacity within the community.

Example: Greater Portsmouth Youth Wellness Coalition

The Greater Portsmouth Youth Wellness Coalition mobilizes and connects the community of Portsmouth, New Hampshire, to improve youth well-being and reduce substance use through prevention activities, health promotion, and resource sharing. In doing so, the GYPWC engages youth in prevention and early intervention programming that address the conditions in which they live, work, learn, and play.

Under the guidance of the Greater Portsmouth Youth Wellness Coalition, several programs have been implemented to support regional youth. The B3 Youth Clinic program in Portsmouth, for example, is a basketball clinic for youngsters at a local playground. The leader of this program, Eli George, is a seventeen-year-old junior from Portsmouth High School. Eli has gathered a group of varsity basketball players from Portsmouth High to offer their services for younger kids. During a podcast interview, Eli said: "From my love for basketball, I wanted to replicate for other kids in the community the feeling that I get when I play basketball, and that's just being able to be yourself and have fun with others without worrying about the stresses of school or work or what's all going on your family. Just being able to leave it out on the court and just have a good time. And so, I wanted a connection."[147]

When asked why he thought community connections were a good thing, he replied, "Because I think when we stop having connections, it usually doesn't end well." Today the program has been operational for two months with an average of twenty-five to thirty kids of all ages showing up for basic basketball skills, scrimmages and just a place to be with our kids sharing a common interest.

Phase 3: Planning

We have now identified enough capacity within the community to get things done. What are our priorities? What should we focus on first? How do we operate as a coalition? What is the action plan and how will it be coordinated?

During the planning cycle we find what works and what is the best way to pursue the coalition's objectives. We dive into the coalition's inputs, the actions, resources, and desired outcomes in a visual manner. Gantt charts, workflow diagrams, and logic models are useful tools to visually understand the interconnection of effort and outcome.

Example: Using a Logic Model

A logic model is a graphic depiction (roadmap) that presents the shared relationships among the resources, activities, outputs, and outcomes/impacts for the program. It depicts the relationship between the program's activities and its intended effects, in an implicit cause and effect relationship between program elements.[148]

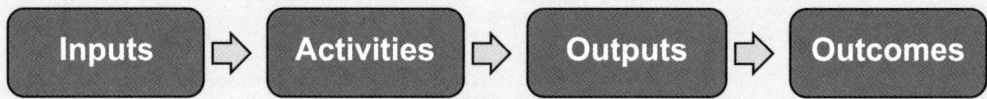

Inputs ⇨ **Activities** ⇨ **Outputs** ⇨ **Outcomes**

Figure 4: Logic Model Flow.

Logic models link program inputs, activities, outputs, and outcomes, mostly in tabular form. Below is an example of a logic model used for the Lewiston-Auburn Recovery Friendly Workplace (RFW) pilot program that I coordinated in 2022 and that is still the planning blueprint for Maine's Statewide RFW program today.[149]

Resources/Inputs	Activities	Program Outputs	Short Term Outcomes	Intermediate Outcomes	Long Term Outcomes
• Pinetree Institute • City of Lewiston • City of Auburn • Strengthen LA • Healthy Androscoggin • Tri-County Mental Health (OPTIONS) • Maine DoL Career Center • Maine DoL Vocational Rehabilitation • Maine Re-Entry Network	• Business engagement & outreach Orientation to initiative • Completion of checklist • Declaration to employees • Resources for employers • Connection to recovery orgs • Policy development & education • Trainings for supervisors • Trainings for employees • Mobilization of RFW champions Engagement of community partners • Collaboration w/ Workforce development • Vocational programming • Recovery coaching • Telephone support • Select companies for the pilot	• Increase # of Letters of Interest • Increase # of RFWs • Increase # of hired employees in recovery • Increased retention rate • 10 national RFW's • Increase # of RFW companies in Lewiston-Auburn • Increased # of business success stories • Increased # of RFW business champions • Resource Guide • Training Offerings • Webinars Series	• Designate 9 RFWs • Improved perceptions and increased knowledge of SUD and stigma • Increased knowledge of resources available to support employees • Increased knowledge and confidence on how businesses to respond to employee concerns • Increased level of engagement among RFWs • Improved workplace morale and satisfaction • Increased willingness to hire people in recovery • Increased access to Narcan • Increased access to recovery resources • Increased business / employee participation in community events and collaborations	• Improved communication in the workplace • Increased company loyalty • Less absenteeism Higher workplace productivity • Increased employee recruitment, hiring & retention • Increased utilization of employee resources • More applicants and/or employees have negative drug screens • Consistent policy change to support recovery friendly principles • Improved participation in workforce development programs • Reduced negative involvement with criminal justice system • Reduced engagement with emergency medical care	• Healthier, more productive employees • Improved workplace culture Healthier communities • Sustained recovery among workforce • Decreased substance use • Decreased overdoses • Decreased negative impacts substance use • Recovery friendly policies become std business practices

Tip: It is useful to begin with the desired outcomes and work backwards to assess the resources/inputs and activities to achieve these outcomes.

Phase 4: Implementation

Implementation is where the rubber hits the road. This is where we put our plans into action and take on the tasks that move the coalition closer to its desired community outcomes. In many situations coalitions deliver evidence-based programming and services to meet the needs of the community, staying true to the plan and being nimble enough to adapt to changes along the way.

It is important to note that during this phase of the coalition, a program coordinator should be tasked with documenting meetings, updating, and distributing minutes, setting up and communicating the coalition meeting agenda, and securely storing documents for record keeping and retrieval. A great example of this phase of the coalition lifecycle is Pinetree Institute's ACEs Master Trainer Program.

Example: Pinetree Institute's ACEs Master Training Program

In October 2018, I was the statewide director of the New Hampshire Works for Recovery program, which was a pilot program funded by the US Department of Labor National Health Emergency to help job seekers in recovery. The grant allowed us to provide funds and programming access to participants so they could receive credentialed training and job placement services. The program also worked with businesses through on-the-job training incentives to hire individuals and families affected by the national opioid crisis.

At that time, I had known Pinetree's executive director, Dr. Larry McCullough, through other channels and we often talked about the growing problem of addiction in southern Maine and Seacoast New Hampshire. It was about that time when Larry approached me about *Resilience*, a documentary that had so moved him that he reached out to two of the principals of the documentary, Dr. Robert Anda and Laura Porter, to ask if he could attend one of their ACEs Master Training events. It was shortly after that trip that Larry and I had our first conversation about ACEs and the impact on downstream health, social, and behavioral issues.

Later that fall 2018, Pinetree Institute sponsored viewings of *Resilience* for small groups of influential leaders from southern Maine and Seacoast New Hampshire. In March 2019, the Portsmouth Music Hall Loft hosted a sold-out viewing of

Resilience. The community conversation about the impact of childhood trauma was growing from a murmur to a buzz.

In May 2019, Pinetree Institute hosted its first Resilience Conference featuring ACEs pioneers Dr. Rob Anda and Laura Porter. A short month later, the Portsmouth Community Coordinated Response to SUD (the origin of the Greater Portsmouth Recovery Coalition) convened to discuss the issue of substance use on the Seacoast. The coalition of more than fifteen city agencies and organizations received seed funding from the city of Portsmouth and Portsmouth Rotary and was charged to address the growing SUD crisis based on trauma-informed principles. The buzz was now a community conversation.

Pinetree hosted the second Resilience Conference in October 2020, which was delayed due to COVID, and therefore held virtually. At the event, Dr. Christina Bethell, a leading author and researcher of positive childhood experiences (PCEs), led a daylong workshop on building positive community responses to trauma. What Pinetree Institute learned from this event was that the conversation was strong, but for the most part restricted to a core set of providers, community-based organizations, and community leaders. The need for more widespread education and awareness beyond conferences was deemed necessary.

Finally, in September 2020, with the country still in a pandemic lockdown, Pinetree Institute hosted a virtual ACEs Awareness Master Trainer Program, led by Dr. Robert Anda and Laura Porter of ACE Interface. Thirty regional volunteers—ten each from eastern Rockingham (New Hampshire), Strafford (New Hampshire), and southern York (Maine) counties—received intensive training to in turn offer ACEs training to their respective communities over a three-year period, and at no cost to the recipients of the training. I was one of the ten trained for eastern Rockingham county. The conversation soon became a roar across the region.

The three regions were intentionally selected due to their proximity to each other, the size and concentration of the populations within the communities, and the relatively high number of supportive services and community-based organizations to train. Collectively our target audience for the three regions were as follows:

- 142 schools

- 40 police departments

- 32 to 38 medical facilities

- More than 820 primary care physicians

- Population of 474,770

As I said to Larry McCullough at that time, it was a target-rich environment. Pinetree Institute's commitment was to provide the three-day training of ACE Interface, a three-year materials license, ongoing support, technical assistance, online resources, and sharing of best practices. For their part, the trainees made the commitment to take part in the full training, average one training presentation per month over a three-year commitment, provide training and support to community champions, and report back following each session. Carolyn Eastman of Pinetree Institute chaired monthly collaboration sessions with the group of thirty master trainers where we shared best practices learned from our individual training sessions.

I was not prepared for the overwhelming success and legacy of that ACEs training program. The final tally of more than twenty-five hundred individuals trained over the three-year program cycle only scratches the surface. Perhaps the most impressive outcome of the program was the fertile ground that was cultivated for the birth of the Greater Portsmouth Youth Wellness Program, which led to a ten-year Drug Free Community Grant, and the Greater Portsmouth Recovery Coalition that has just completed its fifth year of operation.

Phase 5: Evaluation

Evaluation is the process by which outcomes are tracked and coalition programs are measured. The data need to be relevant and causal. It makes little sense to declare that a recovery ready community coalition is going to reduce overdose deaths by X amount. There *may* be a decrease in deaths resulting from a number of factors in the community including, for example, harm reduction; however, it would be exceedingly difficult to draw a cause and effect conclusion that it was the actions of the coalition that led to this outcome.

A more appropriate approach would be to define outcomes that are directly attributed to actions taken by the coalition and its committees. For example, as a result of opening two recovery homes in the community, we've added sixteen beds to the local capacity. Or, as a result of workforce development programs, twenty-five participants have received certificates of training.

Defining Outcomes

Outcomes are an important measure of progress to demonstrate to the community stakeholders, donors, and coalition members to assess progress against coalition goal. Outcomes also provide a diagnostic to determine if other courses of action are better suited for the coalition's efforts. Donors are interested to see if their generosity is being used to effect positive change. The coalition membership will likely appreciate participating in an outcomes-driven program as this provides a view on whether their time investment is making a difference.

- **Team Outcomes:** team outcomes are the result of the Needs Assessment and Planning phases of building the coalition. These outcomes reflect the local goals and intended results. They will likely evolve over time.

- **National Metrics:** national metrics are either or both evidence-based or best practices. An example of a program with national metrics is the National Recovery Friendly Workplace initiative, which is being implemented across the United States, and coordinated by a director of state engagement. At the time of this writing, there is no nationally recognized standard for Recovery Ready Communities. It is recommended that the Recovery Ready Community framework and the minimum elements of a Recovery Ready Community introduced in this book be used as a proxy.

- **Refined Focus:** adapting Team Outcomes to the National Metrics leads to coalition outcomes that are developed locally but guided by a standardized framework.

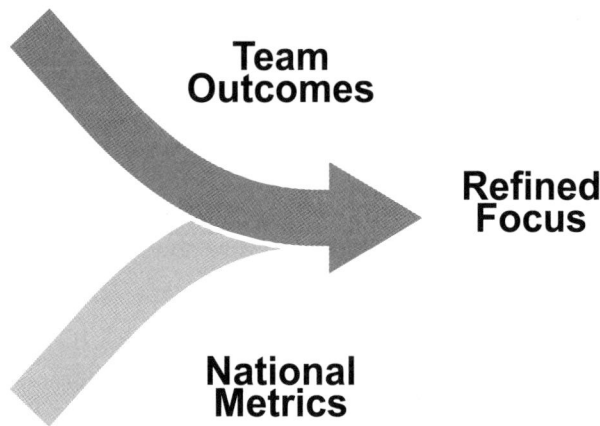

Figure 6: Defining Coalition Outcomes (copyright Pinetree Institute 2024).

The Greater Portsmouth Recovery Coalition outcomes are built upon the groundbreaking work the state of Kentucky did on outcomes. Molly Louison-Semrow explains, "What we did in Portsmouth was to take that scorecard and we adapted it for New Hampshire as there are some state-specific pieces there that just don't apply to our state. We also needed to add things that were specific to us. We've adapted that scorecard with eighty metrics from everything you can think of from corrections to workforce development to the faith community to anti-stigma, recidivism, recurrence, job placement, length of time in a job, etc. We're thinking of giving it kind of a green, yellow, red rating system, something visual. And it's not meant to be a critique per se as to how we're performing. It's more what can we learn from this to do things a bit better and have more of an impact on that."[150]

David Whitesock offers a perspective on defining coalition outcomes as a way to satisfy grant sources: "Governments and counties are the ones dispersing coalition funds. So as a citizen taxpayer, I want to hold that body accountable. Whoever is dispersing that money, I want to hold those people accountable."[151]

Outcomes can be loosely defined during the *Planning* and *Implementation* phases of building a Recovery Ready Community. In the case of the Greater Portsmouth Recovery Coalition, outcomes were refined as the committees and task forces progressed over the *Implementation* phase, and these outcomes reflect the specific work of a given committee, say, for example, harm reduction. During the *Evaluation* phase of the coalition, outcomes were assessed against a specific outcome criteria established over the course of the coalition life cycle. Below is an example of the lifecycle of goals and outcomes for harm reduction using the SAMHSA Strategic Planning Framework.

Phase 1: Assessment: "What are the priorities for addressing addiction within our community?"

Phase 2: Capacity: "We have no harm reduction services in our community."

Phase 3: Planning: "Let's establish a Harm Reduction committee to review options for building capacity."

Phase 4: Implementation: Harm Reduction committee established; Harm Reduction services developed and commence operation in the community.

Phase 5: Evaluation: Outcomes scorecard for Harm Reduction.

Category	Resources/Interventions	Task Force	Notes
Prevention	Safe medication disposal sites/programs	Harm Reduction	Medical disposal at local police departments and select local pharmacies
	NH Harm Reduction Coalition visits sc heduled for the community	Harm Reduction	NH Harm Reduction Coalition visits to Safe Harbor Recovery Center
	Harm Reduction program offers access to vaccinations	Harm Reduction	Families First mobile healthvan visits
	Harm Reduction program offers free HIV and HCV testing	Harm Reduction	NH Harm Reduction Coalition
	Harm Reduction program offers access to free syringe support services	Harm Reduction	NH Harm Reduction Coalition
	Harm Reduction program offers free fentynal test strips	Harm Reduction	NH Harm Reduction Coalition
	Community hosts Naloxone training and distribution	Harm Reduction	NHHRC and Portsmouth Health Department

Table 1: Sample Outcomes Scorecard—Harm Reduction.

Note that it could take years to progress from Phase 1 to Phase 5, as we'll see in the Section 4 Greater Portsmouth Recovery Coalition, where we will provide much more detail across all committees.

Tip: In some communities it may make more sense to start with the definition of desired outcomes and conduct needs assessments based on these outcomes.

Cultural Competence

Within the context of the Strategic Prevention Framework, cultural competence refers to the ability of a coalition to understand and indoctrinate values, lifestyles, traditions, and norms of the community and its individuals. Cultural competence embodies the societal and political leanings into diversity, equity, and inclusion. But cultural competence can and should be so much more than checking a box. It is essential to recognize that recovery supports should be as varied as the people they aim to support. Creating space for individuals to express autonomy and self-determination by identifying and defining their own uniquely diverse journeys with substance use is vital in substance use treatment and recovery support.[152]

Example: Maine Recovery Friendly Workplace (RFW) Statewide Assessment

In January 2022, Pinetree Institute was awarded a grant from the Maine Health Access Foundation to define the requirements and recommendations for a Maine statewide Recovery Friendly Workplace program. The grant was written with specific language that required a Diversity Equity Inclusion (DEI) lens for assessing requirements and making final recommendations.

The feedback we received from underrepresented Maine populations was simultaneously startling and enlightening and has informed all of our work at Pinetree Institute since that study.

A sampling of what we learned:

Indigenous People

- Trauma for indigenous people goes beyond the individual and includes the family and the community.

- Intergenerational loss of identity is in their DNA.

- Recovery Friendly Workplace or any workforce development program needs to address the broader community economic base; create incentives for indigenous people-owned and -managed businesses.

- Educate the community to remove systemic ignorance and lack of education about indigenous issues and culture.

- Bridge the "trust gap"—many indigenous communities are angry at and distrustful of community systems that are perceived as white-privileged.

People of Color or Asian Descent

- Stigma and systemic racism leads to fear for being a person of color or Asian descent in a predominantly white state.

- Systemic barriers in the workforce include hiring practices, promotions, salary, and work assignments.

LGBTQ+ Community

- Stigma in the workplace marginalizes LGBTQ+ workers.

- Members of the LGBTQ+ community don't feel safe in jobs or living in recovery homes unless these operations have LGBTQ+ representation in landlords and management.

- Need LGBTQ friendly wrap-around services.

Justice-Involved

- Need to address the question: does Recovery Friendly Workplace = Felony Friendly Workplace?

- Countless examples of individuals who were in the running for a job, or in some cases *offered* a job, but were denied after background checks revealed criminal history.

- Lack of education for employers and management regarding this untapped labor pool.

- Soft skills and other training are required in many cases.

Women/Women with Children

- Safety as many members of this population are victims of domestic violence.
- Need flexibility regarding paid time off.
- Some have criminal records.
- There exists gender-specific trauma (trafficking, prison, addiction, domestic/sexual violence).
- Lack of transferrable skills.
- Gaps in employment.
- Loss of custody of children.
- Lack of education.

Veterans

- Veterans are typically highly skilled, highly reliable employees—thrive with structure of the workplace such as schedules, teamwork, and meeting commitments.
- Transition from military environment is sometimes challenging, especially if the workplace is casual and free of structure.
- Veterans want to be treated the same as all employees.
- Require wrap-around community and employee services to help with transition to civilian job.

New Mainers (Immigrants, Refugees, Asylum-Seekers)

- Primary needs include housing, integration services, healthcare, education, and jobs.
- Challenges include language, stigma, lack of transferrable skills, fitting in culture-wise.
- Many have experienced existential trauma such as war, famine, environmental disasters, or gang violence.

Taking a step back from the context of this Recovery Friendly Workplace-focused project, these learnings can be applied to any community coalition where such populations live, work, go to school, or try to integrate into the community. Including these folks in the conversation and more importantly, on the coalition will help to ensure that their needs are met and their perspectives are valued.[153]

Spotlight: Equality Community Center, Portland, Maine

The Equity Community Center (ECC) in Portland, ME, is a collaborative workplace for LGBTQ+ and allied social justice-seeking non-profit organizations and has been in operation at its current location at 15 Casco Street since 2021. ECC is a twenty-two thousand square foot office, meeting, and event space, providing a clearinghouse to help members network with the community for the support services they need to thrive. ECC is open weekdays from 9 to 6 and is open to the public. In addition to offering a workspace for meetings and events, the center is the location of Safe Combinations thrift store.

Sustainability

In Chapter 9 we discussed several reasons why building a coalition is difficult. Equally as challenging is sustaining the coalition over time and with the expected turnover of coalition members. Sustainability involves building a system that is effective and adapted in order to achieve defined outcomes.

Washington University in St. Louis offers a Program Sustainability Assessment Tool (PSAT) that allows for a self-assessment of the coalition sustainability against a prescribed set of criteria. The assessment involves forty questions addressing eight domains that can help build the capacity for maintaining a program.[154]

1. **Environmental Support**
   - *What it is*: Having a supportive internal and external climate for your program.
   - *Why it is important*: The ability of the coalition to get things done is dependent on the overall economic and political climate of the community.

2. **Funding Stability**
   - *What it is*: Establishing a consistent financial base for your program.
   - *Why it is important*: Funding cycles put stress on programs and make it difficult to provide consistent quality services, especially when funding sources are not multiyear. Also, programs that rely on a single funding source, rather than multiple sources, are more vulnerable when funding cuts occur.

3. **Partnerships**
   - *What it is*: Cultivating connections between your program and its partners.
   - *Why it is important*: Partners connect the coalition to greater resources or expertise and provide services if your program has to cut back and advocate

on behalf of your cause. Partners can also help rally the community around your program and its goals.

4. **Organizational Capacity**
   - *What it is*: Having the internal support and resources needed to effectively manage your program.
   - *Why it is important*: Organizational capacity encompasses a wide range of capabilities, knowledge, and resources.

5. **Program Evaluation**
   - *What it is*: Assessing your program to inform planning and document results.
   - *Why it is important*: Evaluation helps keep the coalition on track with its goals and outcomes. If evaluation data shows that an activity or strategy isn't working, the coalition can pivot to correct the program's course to become more effective.

6. **Program Adaptation**
   - *What it is*: Taking actions that adapt your program to ensure its ongoing effectiveness.
   - *Why it is important*: Circumstances change and sometimes the coalition needs to as well. The goal is not necessarily to sustain all of a coalition's components over time, but rather to sustain the most effective components and their benefits to the community.

7. **Communications**
   - *What it is*: Strategic communication with partners and the public about your program.
   - *Why it is important*: People need to know what the coalition does and why it's important. Communicating externally about the coalition's effectiveness helps the program gain greater visibility and builds support from partners and the public.

8. **Strategic Planning**
   - *What it is*: Using processes that guide your program's directions, goals, and strategies.
   - *Why it is important*: Strategic planning is the glue that holds sustainability efforts together. Without a strategic direction and long-term goals, programs find themselves only reacting to day-to-day demands. Strategic planning combines elements of all of the sustainability domains into an outcome-oriented

plan. Planning also ensures that the program is well aligned with the larger external and organizational environment.

Other resources for assessing a coalition's sustainability include the Sustainability Self-Assessment Tool developed by the Tamarack Institute. The approach is similar in many ways as the PSAT framework: ten domains organized by People, Process, Resource, and Impact Factors.[155]

CHAPTER 13

PREVENTION

In the next several chapters I will break down each domain of the Recovery Ready Community Continuum of Care into its components. We begin with *Prevention*.

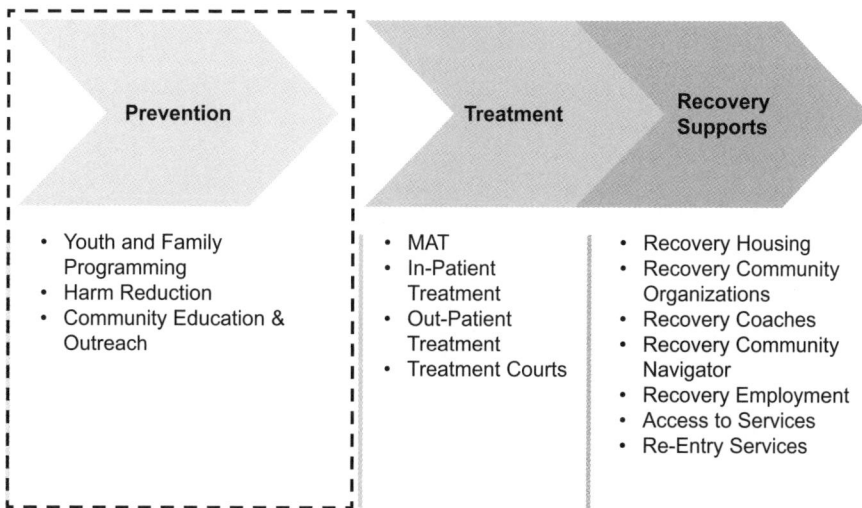

Prevention	Treatment	Recovery Supports
• Youth and Family Programming • Harm Reduction • Community Education & Outreach	• MAT • In-Patient Treatment • Out-Patient Treatment • Treatment Courts	• Recovery Housing • Recovery Community Organizations • Recovery Coaches • Recovery Community Navigator • Recovery Employment • Access to Services • Re-Entry Services

Figure 7: Recovery Ready Community Continuum of Care—Prevention.

In the context of the recovery continuum of care, the national addiction crisis has shown that Treatment and Recovery Support domains alone are not sufficient to reduce the number of overdose deaths, which has surged past one hundred thousand lives in 2022 and 2023.[156] Treatment and Recovery Support interventions mitigate the impact of substance use disorders, but do not necessarily address the root causes of addiction. Although not as tangible in terms of outcomes, Prevention programs and interventions shift our attention upstream in our efforts to prevent substance use in the first place.

"Prevention before the onset of frequent opioid misuse and opioid use disorder is critical to ending the opioid epidemic," stated Drs. Hanno Petras (Pacific Institute for Research and Evaluation) and Zili Sloboda (Applied Prevention Science International) in their publication *Opportunities for School-Based Prevention Strategies Responding to the*

Opioid Epidemic. Their study reveals that in over 66 percent of overdose deaths in 2021, at least one opportunity for intervention existed.[157]

Upstream prevention strategies include mitigating the impact of adverse childhood experiences through programs and relationships that reduce known *risk factors* and promote *protective factors.* These interventions take place where children spend the most time: at home and at school. Applying SAMHSA's Strategic Prevention Framework helps coalitions of caregivers and community-based organizations identify factors that have the greatest preventative impact.[158]

- *Risk factors* are characteristics at the biological, psychological, family, community, or cultural level that precede and are associated with a higher likelihood of negative outcomes.

- *Protective factors* are characteristics associated with a lower likelihood of negative outcomes or that reduce a risk factor's impact. Protective factors may be seen as positive countering events.

Individual-level risk factors include genetic predisposition to substance use disorder or prenatal exposure to substances. Individual-level protective factors include self-image, self-control, or social competence. According to SAMHSA, targeting only one context when addressing a person's risk or protective factors is unlikely to be successful, because people don't exist in isolation. In relationships, risk factors include parents who use drugs and alcohol or who suffer from mental illness, child abuse and maltreatment, and inadequate supervision. In this context, parental involvement is an example of a protective factor. In communities, risk factors include neighborhood poverty and violence. Here, protective factors could include the availability of faith-based resources and after-school activities. In society, risk factors can include norms and laws favorable to substance use, as well as racism and a lack of economic opportunity. Protective factors in this context would include hate crime laws or policies limiting the availability of alcohol.[159]

Prevention strategies, therefore, require both early intervention and interventions that address multiple factors including relationships, communities, and societal scenarios. In the context of a Recovery Ready Community, we'll highlight Youth and Family Programming, Harm Reduction, and Community Education and Outreach as the three domains of prevention within the Recovery Ready Community framework.

Youth and Family Programming

We've learned that prevention begins at home. Preventing childhood trauma (ACEs) in the home and creating positive experiences and meaningful relationships (PCEs) for kids and adolescents as they grow, leads to better health and behavioral outcomes. Youth and family programs are wide in scope and can include national organizations such as the YMCA, 4H, Scouting of America, Little League, or local grassroots organizations in the arts, recreation, and community service.

Prevention programming can also take the form of intervention. For example, youth and family social services that offer behavioral health and substance use disorder services provide support to children, young adults, and families and enable these participants to formally enter a system of care. Examples of such programming are mental health services, age-appropriate intensive programming, group therapy, diversion programs, residential services, and alternative to suspension programs.

Seacoast Youth Services is a nonprofit provider of clinical and support programs for adolescents and youth. Located in Seabrook, New Hampshire, near the northern Massachusetts border, SYS offers a vast array of programming to help kids and their families navigate through behavioral health and SUD challenges.

Sarah Fetras, LCMHC, M.Ed., is a director at SYS and coordinates the Alternative to Suspension program. "So just to give you a little bit of background on that: historically for the past fifteen years or so, SYS ran what we call ASAP, which was the Adolescent Substance Abuse Program, for which Seacoast Youth Services was contracted with a couple of local high schools. If the school had a student with a substance use infraction, that student would get a ten-day suspension. The student, however, could buy back five of those days by attending ASAP. I've had many conversations with our staff around this issue, and we all had this really strong feeling that we shouldn't be suspending kids anymore. It's so counterproductive. How are we still doing this? It's so archaic. We would like to see trauma-informed practices taking place in addition to the idea of restorative justice."[160]

Seacoast Youth Services developed a pilot program in 2024 where instead of students getting sent home, they get bused to the agency. Fetras adds, "There we provide them with programming that is very similar in a lot of ways to what we provide in the Intensive Outpatient Program at SYS. It's set up in the same space. There are some big differences as well, but we're providing them first and foremost with a safe space and supervision. We provide interventions including treatment groups, academic support, and healthy activities to promote mental health. Our philosophy is that sending kids home is not solving the problem, so we created a program that can help kids process what is happening to interfere with their success at school."

The agency saw very positive outcomes. "We're seeing the kids get reconnected and are able to raise their grades. We're seeing that the students learned some skills to be able to navigate their anxiety. We're dealing with a lot of self-regulation, emotional regulation, and other skills that they haven't learned. We're still seeing a lot of post-COVID kids that were in their rooms on their computers and isolated for a couple years, and who had had a really hard time re-entering the school environment. So, we've established relationships with local schools, helping give them a level of support to hopefully create different outcomes for their students."[161]

Example: Chase Home—Community Diversion Program

Since 1877, the Chase Home of Portsmouth, New Hampshire, has been dedicated to providing trauma-informed residential and community-based services to at-risk youth and their families. Their vision is that all youth are able to achieve permanency, which is defined as a safe loving family and home. Chase Home serves youth and families on the Seacoast and from across the state of New Hampshire. The agency provides at-risk youth and families with services and programs designed to address root causes of issues that threaten the family dynamic, stabilization of mental health, and long-term wellbeing and permanency for youth.

In addition to state-mandated programs funded by the New Hampshire Department of Health and Human Services, the organization has expanded some of their programs to increase community access to broader services in an effort to prevent some of the issues that often lead to poor long-term life outcomes. Chase Home offers four programs to a catchment area of seventeen local communities in eastern Rockingham County.

1. **Residential Treatment Services (ages eleven to eighteen):** Wraps customized services around youth who live at Chase Home.

2. **Home-Based Program (all ages):** Clinical and therapeutic services to at-risk youth who are experiencing serious difficulties in their lives; these services are available in the community and inside the homes where youth live with their families.

3. **Seacoast Community Diversion Program (under eighteen)** is an early intervention program that diverts youth between thirteen and eighteen who have committed a chargeable offense from the traditional juvenile justice system.

4. **Independent Living Program (ages eighteen to twenty-one)** assists youth in developing the skills necessary to successfully transition from living at Chase Home—or with their parents in distressed circumstances—into independent living.

To put a human element on the need for these services, within the last year residents brought with them the following experiences prior to entering Chase Home:

- 72 percent experienced physical abuse
- 92 percent experienced emotional abuse
- 52 percent experienced sexual abuse
- 80 percent experienced substance use
- 48 percent required mental health hospitalization
- 88 percent witnessed domestic violence
- 28 percent attempted suicide
- 44 percent participated in self-harm
- 44 percent experienced homelessness

Ashley Murphy is the program coordinator of the Seacoast Community Diversion Program. "The diversion program receives referrals from police departments and Junior Probation and Parole Officers (JPPOs) within the seventeen towns served in Rockingham County for youth who have been charged with a crime. We work with the participants through a customized restorative justice-based contract to repair the harm that has been done as a result of their offense and bring awareness to their actions. Once they successfully complete the program, their charges will be sealed and will no longer be on their juvenile record."[162]

Harm Reduction

Harm reduction generally encompasses an ever-growing suite of strategies that are designed to "meet people who use drugs where they are at, but not leave them there," without any attendant judgment that their continued misuse of opioids constitutes a moral failing.[163]

Harm reduction, also referred to as overdose prevention, is not without controversy. There are some who view harm reduction as enabling drug use. This is not an unreasonable point of view until we look at the science.

Liz Beaude of New Hampshire's Harm Reduction Coalition offers an appropriate response with the data: "In 2022, [Narcan] participants reported that they reversed 1464 overdoses among other participants. Those are 1464 second chances where folks get to go make that second decision about using, they get to see their family or kids again, they get to come back."[164]

So what *does* the science tell us? SAMHSA defines harm reduction as a practical and transformative approach that incorporates community-driven public health strategies—including prevention, risk reduction, and health promotion—to empower people who use drugs (PWUD) and their families with the choice to live healthier, self-directed, and purpose-filled lives.[165]

Harm reduction services can range from the basic (education to reduce stigma), to the comprehensive (fentanyl test strips, distribution of naloxone, syringe service programs), to the medically necessary (wound treatment kits). Harm reduction acknowledges that PWUD deserve the same access to services as those entering a program of treatment and recovery, without stigma or discrimination. Harm reduction spans across the Prevention, Treatment, and Recovery Supports phases of the Recovery Oriented System of Care.

From a public health perspective, harm reduction is critical in reducing the transmission of communicable diseases, such as HIV or hepatitis, which occur when PWUD share needles, pipes, and other drug paraphernalia.

Sampling of harm reduction services:

- **Naloxone:** for reversing an opioid overdose.

- **Fentanyl test strips:** enable people who use drugs to test whether the substance they are using has been mixed or contaminated with fentanyl.

- **Syringe service programs (SSPs):** to prevent the transmission of infectious disease.

- **Safe injection sites:** dedicated spaces where PWUD can use substances under the supervision of trained medical staff. These services can prevent overdose deaths.

- **Wound care kits:** first aid supplies to treat wounds from drug use.

- **Safe sex kits:** to prevent the transmission of infectious disease.

- **Education:** community education and outreach programming to raise the level of knowledge about harm reduction, and to reduce stigma.

Example: New Hampshire Harm Reduction Coalition (NHHRC)

The National Harm Reduction Coalition was founded in 1993 when a small group of activists, educators, and people who use drugs began launching grassroots efforts to support members of their communities who were dying from the brutal disease of addiction.[166] The New Hampshire Harm Reduction Coalition (NHHRC) was established in 2017 by a network of advocates who were engaged in advocating for New Hampshire Senate Bill SB 234 (2017), which allowed operation of syringe service programs (SSPs) in New Hampshire.[167] The coalition was formed in response to the lack of services in the state and addressed that gap by providing essential resources such as syringe services, wound care supplies, and overdose prevention to PWUD.[168]

Today the organization operates thirteen registered syringe service programs across the state of New Hampshire. In addition to harm reduction kits, NHHRC also provides community education in order to help raise the public's understanding of harm reduction and evidence-based practices to prevent overdose deaths and the transmission of infectious diseases.

The coalition uses a nonjudgmental, person-first approach to honor the autonomy and self-determination of their participants and as a means of building mutual respect and trust. NHHRC has recently launched a massive marketing and education campaign under the leadership of Marketing Director Han Hamel. By deploying user-friendly and deeply informative digital and social media marketing techniques, Hamel hopes that the message resonates in a way that addresses the myths about harm reduction, but to also be a catalyst for change. Topics covered include:[169]

- Syringe Services Program

- What is Harm Reduction?

- Help Someone You Care About

- Understanding Fentanyl Test Strips

- Overdose Prevention

- Gender-Affirming Hormone Therapy Guide

- Book our Mobile Services

- Harm Reduction Zines

- Harm Reduction Works Meetings

Spotlight: Compassionate Overdose Reversal

Liz Beaude, NHHRC's director of education and technical assistance, says, "Overdose prevention is not just naloxone going directly into somebody's body, but it includes the steps before a person even experiences an overdose. What we're trying to do in the coalition is move towards compassionate overdose reversal, which everyone would think that's what we're doing anyway, when you're reviving somebody who's having an overdose. But the reality is that when folks are using opioids, and they're having naloxone put into their body, they're just having that opioid removed so quickly from their receptors that they're being put into precipitated withdrawal. And that precipitated withdrawal feels like their bones are melting out of their skin, and they're restless and nauseous and full of every fluid of which you could possibly think. And in that state folks are in such horrific pain that they feel they have to go out and use it again. And a lot of times they're using so much more. They're using without people around them as a safety precaution. And they're telling people 'Do not give me naloxone.' So we try to compassionately reverse these overdoses by being very conscious that people who are getting a lot of naloxone suffer and need to be treated in that moment for acute withdrawal."[170]

Drug Checking Services

The Recovery Research Institute defines drug checking resources as "an approach to harm reduction in which people who use drugs can test the chemicals that make up the drugs they intend to use. This can reveal if the drugs contain harmful substances that the person may not want to consume, such as fentanyl and xylazine, which can substantially increase risk for overdose."[171]

Drug users have a right to know what they are putting in their bodies. Knowledge of potentially lethal ingredients in their drug supply, ingredients that they often had no intent of consuming, can help prevent overdosing, or in this context, drug poisoning. It also empowers people to make an informed decision about their consumption. Examples include fentanyl and xylazine test strips.

Drug Testing Solutions

Drug Testing Solutions offer clinicians the ability to monitor the use of prescription medications and illicit drugs, whereby clinicians are empowered to:[172]

- Monitor and support decisions about medication therapy, particularly controlled substances.
- Identify recent use of prescription medications, non-prescribed medications, and illicit substances.
- Detect medications that may result in drug-drug interactions.

- Advocate for and communicate with patients about individual treatment plans.

- Identify possible illicit drug use and medication misuse or diversion.

Safe Supply Services and Supervised Consumption Sites

In 2022, the Canadian government, in an effort to stem the flow of potentially toxic drugs, implemented a safe supply program in British Columbia with the intent to reduce the risks of drug use and overdose. To that end, the program allowed people who use drugs access to legally regulated drugs in a clinical environment. The safe supply sites offer wrap-around services such as counseling, recovery services, and social workers in the event that a participant chooses to enter into a system of care. It's important to note that entry into a system of care is not a requirement. Initial findings show behavioral and attitude change in consumers of the site, including an increased feeling of dignity and safety. It is too soon to quantitatively measure the outcomes of the program.[173]

Unlike Safe Supply Services, where the regulated drugs are provided to participants, Supervised Consumption Sites allow participants to bring their own supply. Supervised or "Safe" Consumption Services, are designated sites where people can use drugs under the safety and supervision of trained personnel. According to the National Harm Reduction Coalition, over one hundred sites exist in sixty-seven cities in eleven countries around the world. After thirty years of operations, SCS have been demonstrated to prevent overdose, HIV and hepatitis C transmission, injection-related infection, and public disposal of syringes. SCS promote engagement and referrals to other support services, including housing placement and drug treatment.[174]

This approach has its share of detractors, since unregulated drugs from the street continue to support the illicit supply chain of drugs. However, evidence suggests that Safe Consumption Services or Safe Injection Sites are associated with lower overdose mortality, fewer first responder calls for treating overdoses, and a decrease in transmission of infection diseases.[175] Additionally, concerns about these sites leading to increased criminal activity or drug use are not supported by the evidence. One study in Vancouver, Canada, observed an abrupt, persistent decrease in crime after the opening of a supervised injection site.[176]

Community Education & Outreach

Community Education and Outreach often involves a transfer of knowledge or provision of services to populations who may not otherwise have access to them. For example, the current United States Drug Enforcement Administration "One Pill Can Kill" campaign provides the public with knowledge of fentanyl poisoning in the street supply of drugs.

Other campaigns such as the dangers of smoking can run for decades and take a generation or more to have a measurable impact.

Stigma associated with addiction and the impact on individuals and families seeking services is pervasive. Stigma affects one's ability to find work, housing, and other services. Addressing stigma associated with addiction—drug use, treatment, recovery, justice involvement—is a necessary component of a recovery ready community.

Confronting Stigma

Brittany Reichmann is a mother, wife, and beloved champion of the rights of people in recovery. She says, "I have a son, a beautiful baby boy. And he's two and a half years old now. But at around three months, he started experiencing asthmatic symptoms. He was allergic to our cats, and we were going to the emergency room. And at this point, he was having really labored breathing. He had a cold, and we're in the emergency room. And I'm very open about my history. They had my previous notes, which were at the same hospital where I had my son, so they had my medical history, where I disclosed that I was a person in recovery. The ER doctor took what he wanted out of my history. And he relayed to the pulmonologist that I had used while I was pregnant with my son, and it had resulted in major medical complications.

"So we are gone from the hospital, and I have the patient portal app on my phone so I can see the visit notes. So I read all of this the next day. And I was mortified. And I called the medical records at the hospital and demanded that they take these notes out of my son's chart immediately as this could have major consequences for both of us.

"I think of this stigma issue as perhaps being skipped over for a job, even though I know I'm qualified for it. I accept that some of this is a consequence of my addiction and the things that I did during that time when I was using. I am no stranger to the wrongs that I did while I was using and though I might be seven years sober and a completely different person, I hurt people, I hurt institutions, I did things wrong, and some of that is a natural consequence. That was the first time that I was really pissed off for lack of a better term. I was livid."[177]

Sometimes people don't know what they don't know. Stigma can range from an innocent lack of understanding about the facts surrounding addiction to generations carrying the same stereotypes and tropes learned from our family. Education and conversation can address a lack of understanding. I certainly view addiction a lot differently than I did when I was a kid.

When the stigma of addiction impacts our rightful access to basic needs such as housing or employment, the prospects of a person in recovery maintaining that recovery over the long term are diminished. But when stigma impacts our children or other loved ones, it can create a crisis.

In my years of working in the recovery space, I've heard many stories like Brittany's where professionals who should know better, do not. I've sat in a coffee shop in my local community and heard a police officer claim it shouldn't be his job to revive someone who has overdosed, even though he may be the first responder on the scene, and the only person present to save that life. I recognize there is burnout and compassion fatigue. My younger brother retired from a thirty-five-year career as a first responder partly due to his fatigue from reviving the same person multiple times in a week.

Stigma has emerged as one of the most critical barriers facing individuals, families, and communities alike. Fighting stigma takes a lot of time and effort, much like corporations building their brand in the marketplace, the effort takes a relevant message, time, and repetition in order to change hearts and minds. Effective tactics may include media campaigns, podcasts, training, and events.

Rather than hammering home scientific evidence, technical jargon, and black versus white arguments, effective campaigns must meet the audience where they are. There are questions to be heard, fears to be processed, confusion to be addressed.

Education

Community education to address stigma associated with addiction can come in many forms. Formal classroom training, workshops, professional training, social media, and traditional media are all examples of outlets to deliver content and messaging to address stigma.

Pinetree Institute has hosted numerous conferences, workshops, and education programming to help individuals, families and communities build resilience against trauma, mental illness, drug use and the stigma associated with these issues. One of the most impactful programs they offer is the annual Pinetree Institute Resilience Conference, which began in 2019 with Dr. Robert Anda and Laura Porter as keynote speakers on the subject of adverse childhood experiences (ACEs). In 2020, Dr. Christina Bethell was the conference keynote and spoke about the countering effects of positive childhood experiences (PCEs). Follow-on conferences have been held annually addressing topics such as developmental relationships, and resilient communities. Pinetree continues the drumbeat on the impact of ACEs and the promise of PCEs. Pinetree also offers an on-demand Trauma-Informed Certificate Program (TCIP) on developmental relationships and resilience.

Outreach

Community outreach involves establishing a network of community partners and stakeholders for the purpose of communication, knowledge sharing, and perhaps most important, calls to action. A recovery ready community utilizes marketing and media channels to raise awareness of the cause, celebrate successes, recruit coalition membership, and let coalition funders know how their generosity is achieving outcomes.

WSCA, Portsmouth Community Radio (www.wscafm.org), eagerly signed up as the media partner for both the Greater Portsmouth Recovery Coalition and the Greater Portsmouth Youth Wellness Coalition. In this capacity, WSCA offered its facilities for meetings, live programming, and most recently, a twenty-episode podcast series "It Takes A Village: Addiction Prevention & Recovery on the Seacoast." The podcast series chronicles the formation of both coalitions and details about key sector stakeholders. "Help us Get Help" is the tagline for the series and the image used for promotion is a photo taken of a sign that was planted outside the New Hampshire State House during a "die-in" rally in 2014 to create awareness of overdose deaths in New Hampshire.

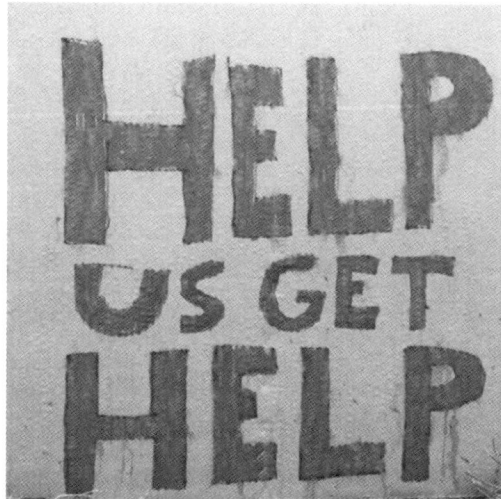

Figure 8: Handmade Sign at New Hampshire State House "Die-In" Rally (photo credit Mark Lefebvre).

CHAPTER 14

TREATMENT

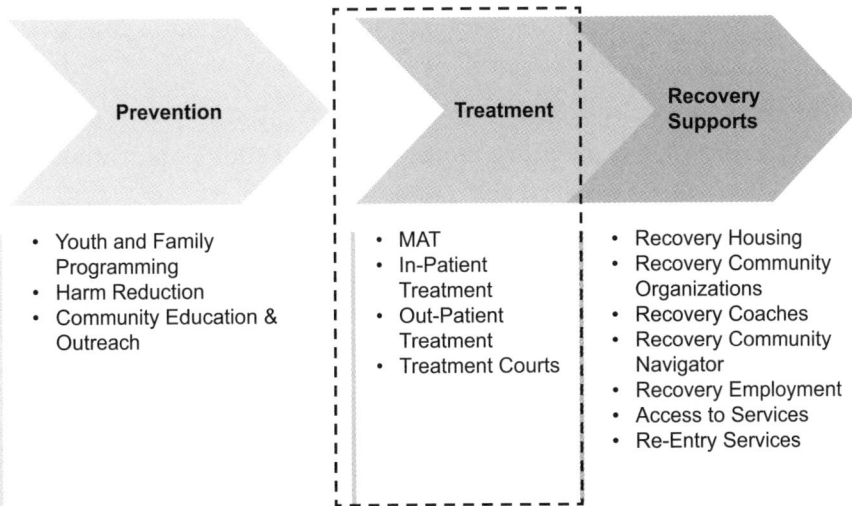

Figure 9: Recovery Ready Community Continuum of Care—Treatment.

Giving Hope to the Hopeless

As I sat on the bed of my bedroom at Michael's House in Palm Springs, California, in August 2012, I believed with every fiber of my being that my life was over. I was crushed by the weight of the consequences of my apparently-not-so-secret life of opioid addiction and alcoholism, and the devastation I laid at the feet of my family back in New Hampshire. Just a few days earlier, my persona was defined as a middle-aged, highly successful executive at a Fortune 50 corporation, dedicated husband and loving father, and a person of high esteem within my community. It was a lie.

My future seemed hopeless. Shame, toxic shame, felt like a heavy blanket. I honestly wished life, my life as I knew it, was over. Then I opened my suitcase and found the cards that my wife Vivian had apparently stuffed in my suitcase.

I read her card first. Despite her shock and anger, she asked me to "fight for her."

The next card I read was from my son, Joey, who was eighteen at the time and about to leave home for his freshman year in college. I recognized his scrawling shorthand as any dad would recognize from his own kid: *Dad, I'm proud that you've taken the steps to get better. I love you.*

The last card was from my sweet daughter Selena, then only sixteen years old and dealing with her own struggles. Her card read: *I just want my old dad back.*

As I collapsed in a heap on my bed, sobbing uncontrollably, I finally arrived at my moment of surrender. In that moment of unspeakable grief, I had the epiphany. Despite all that I did to disrupt their lives, my family, my precious family, was rooting for me. At that moment I made the commitment to them and to myself that I would do anything and everything to recover from the disease of addiction.

That moment was day 1 of my twelve-plus years of continuous sobriety.

The American Society of Addiction Medicine (ASAM) prescribes a multi-level model that is widely accepted as the definitive protocol for adult addiction treatment:[178]

- **Level 4:** Inpatient
  - Medically Managed Inpatient Treatment

- **Level 3:** Residential
  - Clinically Managed Low-Intensity Residential
  - Clinically Managed High-Intensity Residential
  - Medically Managed Residential

- **Level 2:** Intensive Outpatient/HIOP
  - Intensive Outpatient
  - High Intensity Outpatient (HIOP), also referred to as Partial Hospitalization (PHP)
  - Medically Managed Intensive Outpatient

- **Level 1:** Outpatient
  - Long-term Remission Monitoring
  - Outpatient Therapy
  - Medically Managed Outpatient

- **Recovery Residence**

Within the context of this Recovery Ready Community framework, treatment options, whether brick-and-mortar facilities or telehealth services, are not required to exist within the geographical boundaries of the community. Rather, access to these services by transportation or technology is required.

Substance Use Disorder treatment has historically operated separately from general healthcare. Historically speaking, per the US Surgeon General's Report on Alcohol, Drugs, and Health, "with the exception of detoxification in hospital-based settings, virtually all (SUD) treatment was delivered by programs that were geographically, financially, culturally, and organizationally separate from mainstream health care. Of equal historical importance was the decision to focus treatment only on addiction. This left few provisions for detecting or intervening clinically with the far more prevalent cases of early-onset, mild, or moderate substance use disorders."[179] This separation of care creates barriers to access to services, disrupts referrals between providers, and complicates the process of seeking insurance coverage for services.

SUD treatment services include prescribed medication, therapy, and other "services designed to enable an individual to reduce or eliminate alcohol and/or other drug use, address associated physical or mental health problems and restore the patient to maximum functional ability."[180] Examples include detoxification, withdrawal management, medication-assisted treatment, in-patient/residential services, intensive outpatient services, and partial hospitalization programs.

Today there are approximately three thousand addiction physicians in the United States. This capacity, however, is insufficient to meet the needs of the tens of millions of people with a substance use disorder.[181] In rural environments, the shortage of available addiction physicians is ever more dire.

One potential solution gaining momentum is to tap into the more than five hundred thousand primary care physicians in the US and to integrate SUD care into mainstream medical practice of screening, case identification, diagnosis, medication-assisted treatment, harm reduction interventions, and treatment (including psychiatric care).[182]

Medication-Assisted Treatment (MAT)

It is estimated that more than two million Americans have an opioid use disorder (OUD), which as a population has a twenty-fold risk of early death due to overdose, infectious diseases, trauma, and suicide. According to the National Academies of Sciences, Engineering, and Medicine, "as with any other disease, medications should not be withheld from people with OUD without sufficient medical justification. Withholding them on ideological or other non-evidence-based grounds is denying people needed medical care."[183]

Today there are three medications approved by the US Food and Drug Administration: buprenorphine, naltrexone, and methadone. Methadone is a synthetic opioid agonist (chemicals that bind to and activate receptors in the brain causing a biological response) that treats withdrawal from opioids. Long-term methadone maintenance has been shown to reduce overdose deaths, transmission of infectious diseases, and criminal behavior associated with drug seeking.

Buprenorphine is a *partial*-agonist in that it binds to the same receptors as morphine, fentanyl, and heroin, but lower in strength. Similarly to methadone, buprenorphine helps reduce withdrawal symptoms and is often used to stabilize a person who uses drugs. Suboxone, which is a commonly prescribed MAT, falls under the category of buprenorphine.

Naltrexone is different than buprenorphine and methadone in that it acts as an *antagonist* whereby it binds and blocks opioid receptors, and therefore prevents any opioid drug from producing the rewarding effect of opioids. Typically, naltrexone is administered by injection monthly and is regarded as a maintenance medication for Opioid Use Disorder.

People with OUD are less likely to die when they are in long-term treatment with methadone or buprenorphine than when they are untreated. According to the National Academies of Sciences, Engineering, and Medicine, evidence overwhelmingly suggests that "medication-assisted treatment for an indefinite period of time is the safest option for treating opioid use disorder. Treatment using agonist medication is associated with an estimated mortality reduction of approximately 50 percent among people with OUD."[184]

The use of MAT, however, is misunderstood and there is significant stigma as detractors claim that we're replacing the use of one drug with another. According to Dr. H. Westley Clark and Matthew Davis, BS, "From a public health perspective, medications for Opioid Use Disorder are not used often enough because they are under-prescribed by clinicians, whether in primary or specialty care. Stigma, both from the patient and the provider community, coupled with a lack of experience working with people who use drugs, are leading factors as to why these medications are under-prescribed."[185]

MAT is provided across a wide range of resources across the recovery continuum of care including incarceration, re-entry treatment, detoxification, higher levels of recovery housing, primary and specialty care settings, and inpatient treatment, and as a clinical element of intensive outpatient. MAT is an effective intervention that has been shown to reduce opioid use and opioid disorder-related symptoms, reduce the risk of infectious disease transmission, and criminal behavior associated with drug use. MAT also increases the likelihood that a person will remain in treatment and have a higher likelihood of employment.[186] The lack of Medicaid benefits in some states and for underserved populations (e.g., unhoused and incarcerated individuals) creates a significant barrier to MAT access.

Inpatient Treatment

On the afternoon of August 17, 2012, I arrived at Michael's House in Palms Springs, California, and entered a twenty-eight-day inpatient residential program for co-occurring substance use disorder and mental health program. Upon arrival, I was led to a small room by an intake clinician who took my suitcase (including all medications), asked me to empty my pockets, hand over my phone, and take a seat. My first official act as a patient was to blow a .20 in a breathalyzer. I explained that I drank on the flights from Boston through Phoenix to Palm Springs because "I was anxious." Instead of the eyeroll I expected from the clinician, she shared that the majority of patients coming to Michael's House arrive legally impaired. Compassion duly noted.

The professionals and the program of Michael's House probably saved my life. The facility specialized in treating patients with co-occurring mental health and substance use disorders. At that time, I was physically, mentally, and spiritually broken. I was suicidal. Like most of the twenty-five or so male patients, I was under a watch, which meant overnight counselors came into my room on a regular basis to check on my well-being. For this reason, all patients were required to reside in a separate dorm specifically for detoxification. Depending on the substance, detoxification could take anywhere from three to seven days or even longer if necessary. I was given a red wristband, which meant that I could not leave the facility for any external programming such as visits to the gym, external AA or NA meetings, or the daily early morning hikes. I was so sick during detox that it took three days for me to "graduate" to a yellow wristband, which allowed me to take on-premises walks and attend group therapy. It took nearly a week before I stopped hallucinating in my dreams.

Treatment for Co-Occurring SUD and Mental Disorders

There exist specialized residential treatment facilities for co-occurring substance use disorders and mental disorders. Depending on the time and date of various sources, anywhere between 55 to 65 percent of individuals with mental disorders have a co-occurring substance use disorder. It is estimated that over nine million adults in the United States have co-occurring disorders.[187] In such cases, an integrated treatment model for co-occurring (also known as dual diagnosis) cases are becoming increasingly available across the country.

SAMHSA describes best practice principles of an integrated treatment model that includes the integration of mental health and substance use treatment as a co-occurring disorder. This implies that clinicians are trained to treat both and with different services offered to participants at various stages of the treatment and recovery continuum of care.[188]

There are, however, significant barriers to treating co-occurring disorders. Many providers lack training for co-occurring mental health and substance use disorders. Policies limit the ability to provide an integrated approach through restrictive regulations, organizational constraints, licensure and financial issues. Other impediments include lack of service models for co-occurring disorders, measurement of outcomes, and stigma within the medical ranks.[189]

Detox/Withdrawal Management

Withdrawal from substance and/or especially alcoholism, if not managed in a compassionate and medical environment, can be deadly. From personal experience, I can say that a person in the throes of withdrawal often believes they are going to die. Intense anxiety, fever, body aches, diarrhea, vomiting, sweats, and insomnia are common symptoms.

Medical detox is a set of evidence-based interventions designed to manage withdrawal and reduce the likelihood of side effects and other complications as a person adapts to a drug or alcohol-free state. These interventions can include supportive care from medical professionals as well as medications to alleviate symptoms and minimize withdrawal risks.

According to the National Institutes of Health, *inpatient hospitalization* includes around-the-clock treatment and supervision by a multidisciplinary staff that emphasizes medical management of detoxification or other medical and psychiatric crises, usually for a short period of time.[190]

Residential Treatment

Residential treatment for a dual diagnosis of co-occurring SUD and mental disorders often include a combination of pharmacological, psychological, educational, and social mechanisms, in both individual and group settings. Programming is sometimes on a twenty-eight-day rotational schedule with many patients "graduating" to intensive outpatient (IOP) or partial hospitalization programs. Better long-term outcomes are often associated with a transition from a twenty-eight-day residential program to a twenty-eight-day IOP, which helps the individual to ease their way into their job, their family, and their community.

Outpatient Treatment

Intensive Outpatient

Attending an Intensive Outpatient Program (IOP) allows you to continue your treatment plan while moving forward in your life. Addiction Recovery Services offers IOP, but we also allow flexibility that suits those attending school or continuing to work. Here is how our intensive outpatient treatment works.

IOP programs combine group therapy and other therapies for two to four hours during the day or evening. Often, this program occurs four days a week, teaching participants skills that will help them along the journey to recovery. These skills come from cognitive behavioral therapy (CBT) and dialectical behavior therapy (DBT). IOP occurs in a peer setting that will provide participants an opportunity to gain a support system to help achieve their recovery goals.

People who wish to continue working or living at home while in treatment will have that flexibility with an IOP program. People like me, who have returned from an inpatient or residential program, are also candidates for an IOP. I attended two twenty-eight-day IOPs concurrently after leaving in-patient treatment.

IOP programs like those at Michael's House or closer to home at Addiction Recovery Services in Greenland, New Hampshire, typically involve a combination of group check-in, goal-setting for the day, psych education, and process group learning based on a variety of rotating topics. The program is usually facilitated by a master's-level licensed therapist. The process group offerings can vary depending on the patient population but usually includes topics on relapse prevention, healthy relationships, family and recovery, and tools for dealing with anxiety and depression.

Families are regularly updated and involved in discharge planning throughout the patient's participation in outpatient services. Family sessions are arranged by the patient and therapist and can take place in person or over the phone. In some programs, alumni are encouraged to participate, at no cost, in a weekly or monthly process group.

Partial Hospitalization Programs (PHP)

Partial Hospitalization Programs offer a more intensive level of care than IOPs. Typically, PHP-level programs offers six hours of treatment each day, Monday through Friday, and includes weekly individual therapy, daily group therapy, recovery education, holistic activities, aftercare planning, and notably, detoxification.

Partial hospitalization programs offer patients a safe and comfortable way to detox from addiction. Patients in a PHP are closely monitored by medical staff, and the detox process is typically much more comfortable than it would be in an inpatient setting. Additionally, PHPs provide patients with access to individual and group therapy and medication management. This combination of services allows patients to detox safely and comfortably while receiving the support they need to recover from addiction.

Benefits of participating in a PHP program include developing healthy coping skills and tools to build a strong support network at home and in the community and preparing for transition back to everyday life.

Home-Based Treatment

In-home treatment affords the individual and family the option of receiving SUD treatment services within the confines of their home. Aware Recovery Care is perhaps one of the best known examples of an agency that provides in-home services, and operates in eleven states, including the New England states of Massachusetts, Connecticut, Rhode Island, Maine, and New Hampshire. The agency offers a full continuum of treatments including psychiatric services, medicated-assisted treatment, peer coaching, and therapy.

Telehealth/Telerecovery/Teletreatment

Teleservices offer an opportunity to reach individuals and families remotely, which is a benefit for areas of the country that are more remote. Teleservices also provides access to individuals or families that are unhoused.

Example: Better Life Partners

Laura Pratt is senior director for the New England region at Better Life Partners. She shared her experiences serving the state of Maine.

"I should start with saying we are a harm reduction organization, and our focus is very much providing care to underserved populations. For example, by underserved, we mean people that maybe don't have any insurance, or maybe they don't have the funds to get into treatment, or they don't have a car, and they live in rural areas of Maine. They don't have any access to get them to support. So we are trying to focus on that population that's kind of fallen through the cracks. We're able to help them, support them from wherever they are, whether they're living in a hotel room or their home. We even have people living in tent communities around the state. But right now we have a team of five of us that are literally running around the state and going to organizations, going to encampments, going to wherever the need is, and letting them know about our services."[191]

What services does Better Life Partners provide?

"We have a bunch of different options for treatment, and so it's not a one size fits all. We very much put the person in the driver's seat and ask them what they want their recovery to look like. So for substance use disorder, we have what we call addiction therapy or group counseling, where they meet with each other weekly for one hour with a clinical therapist for a therapy session. As you progress in your treatment, the appointments become less frequent, and then it's up to the participant. We also offer medication-assisted treatment for both alcohol and opioid use disorder."

How does the telehealth model work?

"The telehealth option is really helpful because a lot of these people don't have transportation. A lot of them have driving under the influence (DUI) offenses and have lost their license. They don't have the money to pay for a car, and so they're in this place where they can't access treatment. As long as they have the ability to get a phone or share a phone from somebody, we can start with them there. They meet with our doctors via phone, and they have a medical assessment. We see where they're at, what their needs are. We connect them with other community resources. If they're in our program for SUD, they also can access our behavioral health services. So, if they have an underlying mental health condition and they need prescription for anxiety or depression, we can help. We also treat hepatitis C or other infectious diseases."

How do patients pay for Better Life Partners services?

"We take all insurances, and we also treat patients who have no insurance. If somebody doesn't have insurance, we still accept them, we get them on board with us. We get them treatment, whatever they need. And then they will work with one of our counselors down the line, once they're stabilized and in a good place, and then we'll work with them to get MaineCare or state insurance. We turn nobody away."

Treatment Courts

According to All Rise, a national organization that provides membership services, training, and advocacy for justice innovation, treatment courts are considered the most successful justice intervention for people with substance use and mental health disorders. For three decades, treatment courts have proven that a combination of treatment and compassion can lead people with substance use and/or mental health disorders into lives of stability, health, and recovery.[192]

Treatment court (also known as drug court or recovery court), is a public health approach to justice reform in which treatment providers ensure individuals before the courts receive personalized, evidence-based treatment in lieu of incarceration. Treatment court teams are comprised of case managers, law enforcement, community supervision, defense counsel, prosecution, and the judge to provide ongoing support and recovery services to participants.

The statistics tell the story of the success of this approach:[193]

- Over four thousand treatment courts are in operation in the US today.

- Over one hundred and fifty thousand individuals are served by treatment courts per year in the US.

- 58 percent reduction in crime.

- Average of six thousand tax dollars saved per participant.

Judge Tina Nadeau, chief justice (retired) of New Hampshire's Superior Court, served twenty-seven years on the court, and has been a tireless advocate of the New Hampshire Treatment Courts. Judge Nadeau has also been a founding member of the Greater Portsmouth Recovery Coalition, sitting on its steering committee and co-chairing the Recovery Housing Task Force.

"In New Hampshire we consider people who have struggled for a lifetime with substance use and mental health issues. They have lengthy criminal records, including felonies. And the traditional criminal justice response is to say, we've tried probation, we've tried suspended sentences, we've tried house of corrections sentences, and now it's time for you to go to prison. That approach hasn't worked. I've been doing this for a very long time. And if jails and prisons changed behavior, they would be empty. I began to appreciate that we keep applying the same criminal justice response to people and expecting them to change their behavior, but we're not doing anything to give them the tools to change that behavior. What treatment court does is it takes people that might otherwise be headed to the state prison, and we say to them, you are going to get a suspended sentence. But for the first two years, you must be engaged in treatment court. And that's no small task. I've had nearly every graduate tell me that serving two years or so at the prison is a lot easier than completing treatment court. That is because in treatment court participants attend group treatment three days a week for three hours a day, they attend individual counseling at least once or twice a week, they participate in case management meetings once or twice a week, they show up for probation meetings, they submit to random drug testing every single day, they appear in court once a week to tell the judge how they're doing. In summary, they are constantly supervised, and they are constantly working to understand substance use disorder and how to change their behavior. In addition, participants learn evidence-based skills that actually work to rewire their brains. They practice those skills in the community with responses from treatment professionals who can continue to guide them along that path."[194]

Participants in treatment courts face significant barriers including stigma, lack of housing, employment, and lack of access to services. Judge Nadeau concurs. "My experience has been that housing is a major issue, and the lack of recovery homes in particular that are open to taking people with criminal backgrounds that provide the necessary services in the community to support the individual and recovery."

Cheryll Andrews, executive director of Dismas Home, a clinical recovery home in Manchester, New Hampshire, for justice-involved women, is working hard to meet the demand for housing. "The beautiful thing about the treatment court system is that because they have a potential participant ready to begin the treatment court program, we might get a call from one of the coordinators or case managers asking us if we have open beds. Treatment court would really like them to come into our program, and the conversation begins with an application from the participant."[195]

Housing needs go beyond finding brick-and-mortar recovery homes. Judge Nadeau says, "Participants often need money for the first month's rent and last month's rent. We were able to secure funding from the Governor's Commission on Alcohol and other Drugs for bridge-housing assistance to cover those types of expenses, and the support works to improve treatment court outcomes. For example, we had a participant who had back surgery and wasn't getting any disability payment from employment. We were able to use bridge-housing funds to pay for his rent for a couple of months while he recovered. Some people, depending on their level of recovery, need sober living; some people can manage an apartment because they're further along in their recovery. Some people are just starting, so they need emergency shelter while they get stabilized. But in general, housing is probably the biggest barrier, especially for people coming out of jail."

Where do you find the landlords?

"We had one of the greatest housing coordinators, Rachel Azotea. Rachel decided that she would start cold calling landlords all around the state and educating them about treatment court and getting them to understand that people who are in treatment court are highly supervised and likely to be good tenants. The participants are motivated to turn their lives around. If they trip up, they have a probation officer and case manager to support them. As a result, Rachel was able to establish relationships with landlords in various counties and help establish housing options for the treatment court population."

Within the Greater Portsmouth Recovery Coalition, we helped to address the other barriers such as employment through coalition members from Working Fields, Recovery Friendly Workplace, Job Launch, and the New Hampshire Works for Recovery Program. For access to services, we implemented Seacoast Health Connect, a program whereby free (courtesy of T-Mobile) smartphones with prepaid data plans (courtesy of Seacoast Public Health Network), were made available to qualified participants who lacked access to telehealth and telerecovery services. These services are covered in Section 4.

CHAPTER 15

RECOVERY SUPPORTS

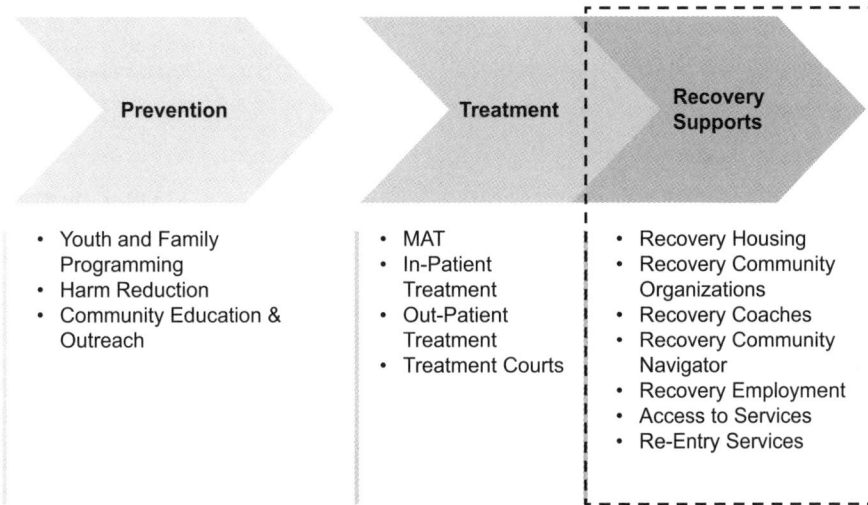

Prevention	Treatment	Recovery Supports
• Youth and Family Programming • Harm Reduction • Community Education & Outreach	• MAT • In-Patient Treatment • Out-Patient Treatment • Treatment Courts	• Recovery Housing • Recovery Community Organizations • Recovery Coaches • Recovery Community Navigator • Recovery Employment • Access to Services • Re-Entry Services

Figure 10: Recovery Ready Community Continuum of Care—Recovery Supports.

Recovery Housing

I have significant lived and professional experiences with recovery housing. When I was discharged from Portsmouth Hospital's Behavioral Health Unit in August 2012, I was told by the discharge case worker that there were no recovery housing beds in the entire state of New Hampshire. When I left Michael's House residential treatment center in Palm Springs in September 2012, there were several houses in various levels of livability to choose from in the surrounding desert communities. The home I selected was the Palm Tee sober living home, a converted motel on the main drag leading out of downtown Palm Springs, and less than a mile away from the twenty-eight-day Intensive Outpatient Program that I attended. It was not a positive experience.

The home was owned by former A&E *Intervention* television personality Ken Seeley, who owned other properties at the time and has since expanded his business significantly under the Ken Seeley Communities brand. At the Palm Tee, the rooms were overcrowded, there was staff turnover, and my two roommates were both using. My roommates were at least twenty years younger than me, and they would often sneak off the premises at night to head downtown to Palm Springs to score. There were no consequences for breaking house rules unless you failed your weekly drug test. Then you were kicked out, typically with your suitcase on the curb and waiting for a taxi. Rarely was there a second chance.

At the age of fifty-four, I was one of the oldest residents. Most of the other twenty or so residents were less than thirty years of age, with a smaller group of older men who seemed to have a longer-term arrangement. My room consisted of three queen-size mattresses sitting on box springs squeezed in about two feet apart. There was no room for any other furniture except for a shared dresser against the wall at the foot of our beds. There was a small closet leading to a shared bathroom.

Each morning we held a house meeting at 6:30 a.m. where there was a roll call that my roommates missed regularly. After a brief 12-step reading from the Big Book of Alcoholics Anonymous, we were off to jobs, IOP, or the gym. On weekends we held a barbeque or did day trips to area attractions. I hiked the mountains and canyons of the desert almost daily.

I share this experience to contrast against today's typical recovery house (also known as sober houses, recovery homes and sober homes). For me, the experience was humbling and humiliating. Fortunately, Palm Springs had been and continues to be a destination locale for treatment and recovery. The Betty Ford Clinic, Hazelden, Michael's House, and countless other providers and hundreds of 12-step meetings (AA, Narcotics Anonymous) were located in the greater Palm Springs area, so I was able to find the help I needed.

Today, there are national (NARR, the National Alliance for Recovery Residences) and state (e.g., MARR, the Maine Alliance of Recovery Residences) coalitions that provide standards for varying levels of care for Recovery Homes. Certification of compliance to these standards is often a condition for opening a home by potential operators.

In the case of the state of Maine, MARR provides organizational support and knowledge-based resources to operators of recovery residences and assists operators in their efforts to comply with state standards and codes of ethics. MARR-certified homes offer a wide variety of recovery pathways including abstinence-based, SMART recovery, and religion affiliated. Most MARR-certified homes allow the use of medication-assisted treatment (MAT) for residents.[196]

Why the need for recovery housing? Recovery homes have been shown to be successful in providing the connection to the community that is necessary for people seeking recovery from substance use disorder. For a disease that creates isolation, shame, and stigma, recovery housing provides a safe environment from which residents can seek employment, attend outpatient programs, and build coping skills to benefit them as they rebuild their lives.

NARR specifies four types of recovery residences[197]:

1. **Level 1 (Type P):** Peer-run, decisions made solely by residents; illicit drug/alcohol free; maintains a recovery-supportive culture and community using house rules and peer accountability.

2. **Level 2 (Type M):** Managed environment, illicit drug/alcohol free, house rules, appointed resident leader, peer accountability; senior residents often appointed as house manager.

3. **Level 3 (Type S):** Supervised activities, illicit drug/alcohol-free, staffing, life skills programming, recovery planning, intended for populations requiring more intensive support than Levels 1 or 2.

4. **Level 4 (Type C):** Clinical services provided, illicit drug/alcohol free integrates social and medical with a combination of supervised peer and professional staff; many offer licensed treatment programs.

Lack of recovery housing is considered a major reason for recidivism and re-occurrence of drug and/or alcohol use. Unfortunately, there is a nation-wide shortage of recovery housing beds. Medication-Assisted Treatment (MAT) is slowly becoming more accepted for residents who are being treated by a clinician for withdrawal management.

What does a typical day in a quality recovery home look like? Cheryll Andrews says, "At Dismas Home, a resident is up and has visited the med office. By 7:45 she is up and dressed, with her room cleaned and sorted and downstairs for the day by 9:30. Everybody is downstairs for the day between 9:30 and 4:00.

"The week is made up of appointments for healthcare, and other benefits, workforce development, volunteer hours, and group therapies. They might go to an offsite meeting with staff, most likely a community meeting. They participate in equine therapy once a week, a beautiful thing to watch. Residents work with case managers for at least one hour a week. Everyone works together to build a foundation. They're not sitting with nothing to do."[198]

Spotlight: Restoring Dignity—Magnolia House

Magnolia House sits on a country road near the Hampton (New Hampshire) downtown intersection with US Route 1. Passersby would not identify this restored country home as a recovery home. Magnolia House opened in 2020. At the time I was leading the Greater Portsmouth Recovery Coalition; shortly after the opening of Magnolia House, we invited the home's owner, Jules Johnson, to join the Recovery

Housing task force. Up until Magnolia House opened in 2020, there were exactly zero beds in all of Rockingham County, the wealthiest county in the state of New Hampshire.

Jules invited me to meet at Magnolia House. I was not prepared for the overwhelming feeling of comfort as I walked into the kitchen and took in the colonial restoration, the warm colors, and the splash of sun coming in through the living room windows.

I interviewed Jules this past summer on my podcast series to learn more about the process of opening and sustaining a recovery home.

How did Magnolia House come to be?

"I think, in August of 2020, right downtown, I had bought the perfect home with a detached barn. I slept in my car with my dog for a year in a parking lot to save money in order to renovate the barn. And so the irony in all of this is that because I had taken all those sacrifices, I was able to offer up this very large house that is perfect for recovery housing, and I had a place to live at the same time on the same piece of property. I think I opened a month later in early September of 2020."[199]

Why open a sober home?

"I opened Magnolia House as a nonprofit because that just seems like the right thing to do for recovery housing, and it seemed like the right thing to do for women in need. It just made sense. I just strictly went on the notion of what I would want as a human. What would be the healthiest way for me to heal?

"It is a healthy, healing home that isn't stacked with twin beds and bunk beds and furniture that is mismatched. It's not a flophouse. We have matching utensils! I want it to be a home that creates the notion that we're worth this comfort. And we've extended that to the property itself. There is a fire pit. There are bonfires. We have a garden with cucumbers and tomatoes. Our residents do a lot of stuff around the house to keep it up and running and keep it beautiful."

Summerwood House

Based on the success of Magnolia House and the lack of sober living beds for men in the community, Jules and I were in early discussion on how to open a men's house in Hampton in November 2021. What transpired over the next several weeks to make this happen is truly remarkable.

In early December 2021, I was nursing a cold brew iced coffee at Blue Harbor Coffee, a small but vibrant community hotspot, where I fondly tell the owners, Josh Yazgan and Stephanie Bergeron, that "shit gets done." I was approached by a former neighbor and local entrepreneur, Al Fleury, who told me he was interested in developing property for people in recovery. I immediately thought of Jules and our prior conversations. Jules, Al, and I met shortly thereafter at a property a couple of blocks away from Magnolia House, for introductions and for a walkthrough of the building.

Later that same week at a Pinetree team meeting, we were approached by Alan Gold, the president of Pinetree Institute's board of directors, about a meetup with a gentleman who was interested in helping the recovery community, but with the caveat that he was to remain anonymous. We circled back to Jules to see if she could quantify the startup costs for opening the new home at the Fleury property. Jules calculated that she needed funding for renovations, furniture, and fixtures, as well as six months of rent in reserve to cover her expenses as she gradually rented out each bed. The anonymous donor wrote a check for that amount.

In less than two months, what started as a conversation between Jules Johnson and me led to the opening of Summerwood House in early February 2022, a ridiculously short period of time.

I asked Jules what her take was on the opening of Summerwood House.

"As you said, all the stars just aligned one day, and everything just kind of fell into place. I think from conversation to door opening, it was like seven weeks, because we had a conversation before Christmas, and you opened just before February, yeah. And I mean, it was a hard push, but we did it.

"Magnolia House at the time had ten beds, and we had another twelve beds at Summerwood, so we had the first twenty-two beds in all of Rockingham County for that period of time. I think we were able to pivot even better, leaning more into that brand of dignity because of that private donor."

A New Business Model

In 2023, Jules enhanced her business model to focus more on quality of life related outcomes, and less on quantity of beds. The Summerwood House lease was not renewed. The women's program at Magnolia House was phased out and the men from Summerwood House were relocated to Magnolia House. The men who relocated to Magnolia House had built up some significant recovery time. Many were dads. The new model, which is the essence of the Magnolia brand, is reunification with dignity.

"We did a big renovation last year, and with that renovation, we really pivoted, and we intentionally tailored to a brand which would demonstrate quality in home, health, and healing. With compassion and dignity in there, you know. We now have eight single private rooms which allows the dads to have their kids stay."

I asked her, "What about outcomes? How are the men at Magnolia House doing today?"

"One hundred percent of our residents are employed," she said. "Six out of eight guys have their driver's licenses back. Five have their own vehicles parked out back. They get their mail delivered here. One hundred percent have bank accounts. One hundred percent have been reunited with their children and are now co-parenting, which is highly unusual for a recovery home."

I asked her, "The Magnolia House model has developed a reputation for recovery with dignity. How can you grow?"

"Yes, we now established a name for ourselves," she said. "We have a thirty-person or so waiting list. We have a reputation. But residents have to want this. This isn't a crash pad. You're not checking a box. You're gonna have to find a job. You're gonna have to take care of yourself. There are non-negotiable requirements for living here.

"The challenge is funding. In New Hampshire, we literally don't have any state funding. We have no federal funding. At Magnolia House we don't. It's a difficult place to start up without either an angel that comes through or a potential grant that comes through the opioid abatement or other channels within the SUD world."

"Is there a particular community experience that stands out from the others?" I asked her.

"Let me start by saying that dads in recovery are not second-class citizens," Jules said. "But in early recovery, they have nothing. They roll in with nothing.

"In 2022, Christmas was right there, and we're a nonprofit, not much money. You were able to hook us up with Santa Claus, which was Rusty Bridle [former firefighter, town selectman and vice president of the Hampton Area Chamber of Commerce], who is one of the nicest, kindest individuals that I've ever met. Santa brought toys donated by the Hampton Fire Department, and gift cards for the dads from local businesses.

"Rusty consistently shows up for us when we are in need. Recently we needed a newborn child's car seat. Who do I call? Rusty. Where did I pick it up? The Hampton Fire Department.

"And so our community has embraced us. We are able to reunify the dads with their children in a healthy home. This is not a flophouse. We fix two generations of addiction. Daughter gets to learn what a healthy male figure looks like and what his friends look like, and how they can play video games without the use of drugs and alcohol. So that eight-year-old now knows what healthy friendships looks like. So we try to break the transgenerational cycle of childhood trauma, and that's exactly what we do. The guys all have their own bedrooms so they can have their kids sleep over with them."

Recovery Community Organizations (RCOs)

Recovery Community Organizations, which are also sometimes referred to as Recovery Community Centers, are nonprofit organizations, founded and led by members of the local recovery community. RCOs were born out of the need to do more to support people experiencing substance use challenges, and offer community education about addiction and recovery, advocate for fair and equitable public policies, run anti-stigma campaigns, and/or offer no-barrier access to peer-based and other recovery support services.[200]

Because these organizations are typically nonprofit, they rely on funding from grants, foundations, and individual donors to operate. RCOs also rely on community support, and visibility within the community. What good is an RCO if it's tucked away in an obscure section of town where no one knows about its presence?

According to Faces & Voices of Recovery, an RCO is an independent, nonprofit organization led and governed by representatives of local communities of recovery that conducts ongoing local recovery support needs assessment, organizes recovery-focused policy and advocacy activities, and provides peer recovery support within the community. These activities are available to all community members and are not restricted to individuals enrolled in a specific educational, treatment, or residential program. [201]

Recovery Community Centers were exceedingly rare until grassroots efforts at the community level led to a slow, but steadily increasing number of centers opening in the early- to mid-2010s. State agencies and governance bodies eventually developed common practices within their jurisdictions to ensure a common delivery model for recovery services. Early examples of grassroots recovery community organizations include Hope for New Hampshire Recovery (Manchester, est. 1999[202]) and the Recovery Project (Greenfield, Massachusetts, est. 2003[203]).

Spotlight: Building a Recovery Community Organization—Safe Harbor Recovery Center

In 2014, I was required to complete a project as part of my graduate studies at Southern New Hampshire University. At that time I was studying for my master's degree in Community Mental Health and Substance Abuse. My project was on the subject of Healing Circles, a practice of indigenous communities for crisis resolution. While doing research for this project, I experienced a profound epiphany that perhaps a peer recovery model could help address addiction in the Portsmouth community.

Safe Harbor Recovery Center of Portsmouth, which opened in spring 2016, was born out of this project when I, my wife Vivian, and Sandi Coyle, a member of the local recovery community, built a coalition of like-minded volunteers to conceptualize, raise money for, and ultimately open for service in the West End of Portsmouth, New Hampshire.

- We held events to build coalition membership including in our homes and at convenient community locations such as the local community radio station, the public library, and other community spaces.

- We scheduled meetings with the mayor and city department heads to build political support.

- We met with and compared notes with Hope for New Hampshire Recovery, which was another recovery community center in its early days of operation.

- We met with a small group of investors and business leaders for building a network of potential donors.

- We held the first of several donor events at a local theatre with compelling guest speakers.

- We conducted outreach to our local newspaper for a number of stories.

The center today offers a wide variety of services to individuals and families including recovery meetings, employment services, services for the homeless, transportation in the form of bus tickets, and referrals to other community organizations.

Today, Safe Harbor Recovery Center is a founding member of both of the Greater Portsmouth Recovery Coalition and Greater Portsmouth Youth Wellness Coalition and continues to provide direct services and programming to support individuals, families, and community members. A few of the notable programs include Job Launch workforce development; distribution of harm reduction supplies; hosting of mutual aid meetings such as Alcoholics Anonymous, Narcotics Anonymous, and SMART Recovery; and innovative programming such as the Alternative Peer Group, oriented towards youth populations. They also deliver supplies to unhoused people and families across the Seacoast.

RCO Programming

SOS Recovery Community Organization in Dover, Rochester, and Exeter, New Hampshire is a nationally accredited RCO and offers what I consider to be the most impactful RCO in the state of New Hampshire. A sampling of SOS's robust array of service offerings:[204]

- Advocacy
- Telephone Recovery Support

- Recovery Support Services

- Family Recovery Programs

- Criminal Justice Recovery Programs

- Harm Reduction Services

- Recovery Friendly Workplace

- Parenting Programs

- Training

SOS also stages an annual two-day conference entitled R.I.C.H. (Recovery-Inclusion-Community-Harm Reduction) that is typically attended by hundreds of attendees and exhibitors.

RCO Outcomes

Outcomes matter for RCOs just like they matter for any provider or community-based organization. Target outcomes vary from one RCO to another. In 2023, Safe Harbor Recovery Center achieved the following outcomes:[205]

- 1,495 people served

- 1,432 people received peer-led services

- 1,290 people received wellness services

- 72 participants overcame health barriers and became "work-ready"

- 29 participants gained jobs

Portland Recovery Community Center (PRCC) opened its doors in 2012 as a small recovery community center on Forest Avenue in the southeast area of Portland with just three staff members. Like many ROCs in the early 2010s, PRCC was part of the grass-roots effort to open recovery community centers nationwide. The organization's initial focus was to build and offer recovery assets to assist the individual and family seeking recovery services. During this time, PRCC developed a robust array of support groups, social activities, and peer support services, including Telephone Recovery Support (TRS) services and Recovery Coaching.

PRCC became an independent nonprofit in 2017. Governed by a volunteer board of directors whose membership includes a majority of people in recovery, the board also includes family members and friends who identify as recovery allies.

In 2017, the newly formed board of directors embraced a bold vision to help make recovery community centers available in every community in Maine. PRCC was awarded a state grant to create the Maine Recovery Hub in order to raise the RCO capacity across the state.

In 2018, PRCC began its work as the Maine Recovery Hub, and today there are twenty-one recovery community centers in Maine with PRCC providing support, training, and technical assistance to these centers. The Recovery Hub has trained well over seven hundred peer recovery coaches and founded the Maine Recovery Coach Certification Board, now an independent certifying body for peer recovery coaches statewide.

In 2021, PRCC purchased and moved into its current location, a new building at 102 Bishop Street in Portland. The building is twice as large as its previous home. PRCC is a nationally accredited RCO.[206]

Portland Recovery Community Center executive director Leslie Clark said, "In the recovery community center model, everything is peer based. At PRCC, we offer three program categories of peer support, advocacy, and education in communities."[207]

I asked her to tell me more about the peer model at PRCC.

"I think that it is really important that RCOs accept multiple pathways and that everything is peer-based," Clark said. "At PRCC, everything is peer-based. We have an average of between 125 and 150 volunteers in any given month. We do a volunteer orientation every Tuesday morning. Sometimes there's a couple of people in there, sometimes there's ten people in there. But we rely on volunteers, greetings at the front door, the front desk, making the coffee, everything is volunteer-driven.

"If a person walked in the door of PRCC and they're looking for help to recover from substance use, a peer member is there to welcome them, asking them where they are, but sharing our own journey. We've all experienced the depths of despair they are maybe experiencing. That's the power of peer."

I asked her, "How do you work with other communities about opening a recovery community organization under the Recovery Hub model in Maine?"

"We'll talk with a group who wants to start a recovery community organization in their town. We ask a lot of questions and explain, here's what we did, here's how it worked for us, and we'll share anything and everything, just like we do with an individual in recovery. So we approach it in that same open way. We share some of the mistakes we made along the way, like, you know, where we screwed up, or where we're still learning, or what we don't know, all those kinds of things. Who helped us? Where did we get help? So it's just taking peer recovery to the macro level."

Clark went on, "For those recovery community centers already up and running, we offer support and trainings on best practice standards. We continue to offer training and continuing education. We bring all the RCO managers together on a regular basis to do training, but also to find out what's going on with them, and connect and collaborate on projects, training coaches, recovery coaches, etc."

"What about the role of advocacy?" I asked.

"That's the second arm of our role as recovery advocates. I think the RCOs in any community are the heart of that community. The center provides outreach through our member ambassadors, such that we have a cadre of people who can go to rotary club meetings or go speak at a church or go testify before the legislature as we move into advocacy. What do people need in their community, and how do we as a community of people who are in recovery ourselves effectively advocate for what we need."

"For too long, and I personally experienced being a nonprofit leader who did not share that I was in recovery for the first twenty-seven years or so, but as we were in the midst of the opioid crisis, I came to realize that if our voices were not at the table, these decisions about policy and funding were being made by well-intentioned people, but in some ways, who didn't understand our needs."

And what about education in the community?

"Part of the role as the recovery hub is to provide the trainings, the continuing education to Peer Recovery Coaches," Clark said. "PRCC conducts statewide training of peer recovery coaches, and I believe we are now well over seven hundred coaches that we've now trained in Maine. We also started Maine's Peer Recovery Coach Certification Board, which registers and certifies recovery coaches. We host a regular meeting of recovery coaches, and we provide culture vision, which is the CCAR (Connecticut Community for Addiction and Recovery) peer supervision model."

I asked her, "What have you learned?"

"Avoid mission drift. For example, I think keeping mission and best practices for the recovery community center model [should be] top of mind and in the forefront of our operation, especially in our role as the hub. All the different centers, we experience this pull or this push to be something different. There may be an urgent community need. Or say the RCO is in a small rural community, and there isn't a food bank, or there isn't a homeless shelter, and you've got people coming in that aren't necessarily seeking recovery. They are looking for food. They're looking for a pair of shoes, a pair of boots. They're looking for a place to sleep. And because no one else in that community is meeting the need, they start to drift in their mission. And it's a tension. So beware of mission drift."

Even in rural communities where those social services may not exist?

"I remember this article that was all about, beware of mission drift, don't start a clothing closet, basically. Well, that might work in Portland, because we do have partner agencies where we can refer people to. But, if you're a small community center where you have a staff of one person and a couple of volunteers and a situation arises for social support, if they're not at the center because they are taking food to someone's house, what does that say about the center's mission? It is really easy to lose what you're supposed to be doing, which takes a huge amount of effort and building your community of recovery people. And so I think mission drift and not sticking to the ten best practices of a recovery community organization is a huge pressure on some centers."

Recovery Coaches

Peer recovery coaches, or simply recovery coaches, provide a valuable service to the community as volunteers and paid staff at community-based organizations and service providers. Peer recovery coaches are sometimes staffed and trained by Recovery Community Organizations for programming within the RCO, and for providing peer services to other partners within the community such as jails, hospitals, and support employees at local businesses. Recovery coaches are effective as they lower the perceived power differential between the coach and person seeking recovery support. They've "walked the walk," and sometimes have very similar life experiences as the person seeking help.

In New Hampshire, Certified Recovery Support Workers, or CRSWs, receive a minimum of fifty-eight hours of classroom or online training on a number of topics including Recovery Coach Academy, Ethical Considerations, Suicide Prevention, and HIV/AIDS & Other Infectious Disease Training. There are electives available including Motivational Interviewing. CRSWs in training must complete five hundred hours of volunteer or paid work under clinical supervision and then take an exam prior to applying for certification. I became certified as a New Hampshire CRSW in 2017.

Recovery Community Navigators

A Recovery Navigator Program provides community-based outreach, conducts intake, and needs assessment, and provides connection to services for individuals and families dealing with substance use disorders. Services may include case management, recovery coaching services, and referrals to a broad range of community resources for mental, behavioral, or substance use disorders. These navigators can be crucial in connecting individuals to recovery resources, offering support in the form of (non-clinical) peer counseling, and bridging gaps between people in recovery and community resources like housing and healthcare.

The role of a Recovery Community Navigator is largely an unmet need within New Hampshire and Maine. Leslie Clark of PRCC believes this role would be a good fit for the RCO. "Think of somebody who is community-based, who understands all of these resources, and who can help somebody get to the help that they need when they need that help. It happens so much within an RCO, people are coming in, or family members calling in, and we're helping them connect to those resources.

"A Recovery Ready Community is a network of coordinated services along a continuum for people to get what they need such as treatment, harm reduction, recovery, support services, housing, all those kinds of things. But a network of coordinated services that a community would need to have, to be able to say they're recovery ready, all those same elements, work, housing, everything, transportation, treatment, the RCO is really acting as the hub of a Recovery Ready Community. So it's where all of these elements come together. It's where we guide individuals and their families throughout their whole journey."[208]

Recovery Employment

Addiction has a profound effect on the workplace. According to the Federal Recovery-Ready Workplace Interagency Workgroup, in 2021, 26.9 million Americans aged eighteen or older with a substance use disorder were employed. Of these, 77.6 percent (20.9 million) were employed full-time. Employers are both especially hard hit by substance use disorder and uniquely positioned to address it in a way that benefits not only them, but their employees, and the broader community. Untreated substance use disorder is extremely costly to employers, resulting in missed workdays, reduced productivity, unnecessary employee turnover, and increased healthcare costs. Substance use disorder can also make hiring qualified candidates challenging and can increase the risk of work-related accidents and associated liabilities.[209]

In a 2017 study completed by PolEcon Research, untreated addiction cost the New Hampshire economy $2.63B per year in lost productivity, up from $1.84B in 2014.[210] Driven largely by the enormous economic impact of addiction in the Granite State, Governor Chris Sununu established the nation's first Recovery Friendly Workplace (RFW) program in the United States in 2018. The program promotes individual wellness for Granite Staters by empowering workplaces to provide support for people recovering from substance use disorders. New Hampshire businesses that become designated as RFWs support their communities by recognizing recovery from substance use disorder as a strength and by being willing to work intentionally with people in recovery. RFWs encourage a healthy and safe environment where employers, employees, and communities can collaborate to create positive change and eliminate barriers for those impacted by addiction.

Also in 2018, the state of New Hampshire was one of five states to receive a three-year demonstration grant from the US Department of Labor to offer training and job placement services for qualified individuals and families impacted by the opioid crisis. The grant, referred to as the National Health Emergency (NHE) grant, encouraged grantee states to test innovative approaches to address the economic and workforce-related impacts of the opioid epidemic.[211] I was hired to direct this program for New Hampshire in October 2018.

The motivation for this program was that the opioid crisis had and continues to impact businesses across the county. Business concerns include difficulty finding qualified workers who could pass drug screens, rising healthcare costs, increased absenteeism, and reduced productivity.

Along with housing and transportation, employment is one of the most critical factors for long-term recovery. Employment reduces recidivism among people involved in the criminal justice system and is associated with enhanced rehabilitative outcomes for the individual and public safety outcomes for the greater community.[212]

There are many obstacles facing individuals in recovery including criminal records, lack of documentation (Social Security, proof of residency, registration for Selective Service for men), lack of transportation, lack of meaningful employment history, lack of skills, and lack of housing. Without government assistance for workforce programming, and without local boots on the ground to provide navigation and case management for job seekers, it is exceedingly difficult for job seekers in recovery to find work. During the Maine Recovery Friendly Workplace program, we interviewed and surveyed a modest number of job seekers in recovery with regards to their fears and concerns:[213]

- How do I deal with my criminal behavior? Should I disclose?
- Lack of confidence and self-esteem
- Lack of education and/or training
- Lack of transportation
- Lack of affordable housing
- Difficulties securing documents (e.g., license, proof of residency)
- Fear of stigma in the workplace
- Lack of childcare
- Need flexible schedule to attend parole meetings, therapist appointment, 12-step meetings.
- Fear of drug screening when on medication-assisted treatment

Additionally, there are legitimate concerns from businesses who express an interest in hiring an individual in recovery, especially if that individual has a criminal record. A sampling of concerns raised as part of the Kennebunk Coordinated Response to SUD:[214]

- Concern about employee relapsing.

- Concern about negatively affecting employee morale and work environment.

- Questionable reliability and trust.

- Concern about theft, erratic behavior, personal appearance.

- Concern about retaliation if the employee had to be let go.

- Concern about undesirable associates of the recovering employee showing up at the workplace.

- Lack of resources and understanding needed to be fully supportive of their recovery process.

The reality is that in a recovery ready community, there is a need for support for job seekers and businesses alike. Programs such as the US Department of Labor National Health Emergency grant, the now-national Recovery Friendly Workplace program, and local grassroots services are filling the void.

In Seacoast New Hampshire, we were very fortunate to have four outstanding programs to address the impact of addiction in the workplace, including the so-called New Hampshire Works for Recovery program that I just referenced. What we found over the course of the early deployment of these programs was that businesses were often confused over which organization and program did what. Although the leaders of the individual programs thought we did not overlap, businesses thought otherwise. We lacked a coordinated message to position these programs and eliminate confusion. What we needed was a coordinated effort.

Example: US Department of Labor National Health Emergency (NHE) Grants

In 2018, the United States Department of Labor awarded five state grants for demonstration projects to address the opioid crisis through employment and training services. New Hampshire was one of the six states and received five million dollars over two years. Other states receiving grants were Alaska, Pennsylvania, Washington, Rhode Island, and Maryland. Maine received this grant in the ensuing grant cycle about a year after New Hampshire.

The grants encouraged states to test innovative approaches to address the economic and workforce-related impacts of the opioid epidemic. Grantees had wide latitude in how the funds could be used, as long as they fell under one or more of the following categories: services for people affected by opioid addiction, their family members, or others living in communities hard hit by the opioid crisis; training for workers to address the crisis; and partnerships and systemwide investments to align workforce services with services provided by other organizations in the community.[215]

The New Hampshire grant was managed by Southern New Hampshire Services, one of the state's largest nonprofit organizations that oversaw community action programming. I was hired in October 2018 as the statewide program director for what was named New Hampshire Works for Recovery.

The three primary goals of the program:

- Test innovative approach to address the economic and workforce-related impacts of the opioid epidemic.

- Provide training and support to dislocated workers, new entrants in the workforce, and incumbent workers, which have been directly or indirectly impacted by the opioid crisis.

- Provide training that builds the skilled workforce in professions that could impact the causes and treatment of the opioid crisis.

With a team of three statewide Career Navigators and three Job Developers, the program provided a pathway to individuals and families impacted by the epidemic, and to identify suitable On-the-Job Training and direct placement opportunities within the business community. The program was operated hand-in-hand with the New Hampshire Recovery Friendly Workplace, which provided additional training and technical assistance to interested employers and their staff. A WorkReadyNH program was developed with the Community College System of New Hampshire to provide "soft skills" training for participants. The curriculum for this program included resume-writing workshops, mock interviews, calendar, email, and other entry-level business practices. Supportive services were funded for qualified participants including short-term rent, transportation, auto repairs, purchase of clothing, childcare reimbursement, and other needs that proved to be a barrier for employment.

Although the program was originally scheduled for a two-year term, a no-cost extension of one year was approved. Nearly three hundred individuals enrolled in the New Hampshire Works for Recovery program with nearly 44 percent receiving credentialed training, 21 percent of participants receiving on-the-job training, 100 percent receiving individualized services, and/or job placement.

Example: Granite Pathways Job Launch

Granite Pathways was founded in 2009 and is a New Hampshire member of the Fedcap Group, an international nonprofit committed to creating opportunities for people with barriers to economic wellbeing. Safe Harbor Recovery Center in Portsmouth, New Hampshire, is a program operating under Granite Pathways.

An example of such a workforce development program is Job Launch, which was launched in 2019, and is a program focused on helping job seekers to build recovery capital—a combination of personal, social, family, and community tools and resources that help participants achieve, sustain recovery, and develop a healthy lifestyle. Employment specialists meet the individual "where they're at" and guide them, via confidential and free one-on-one service, using a comprehensive service plan that is customized to their personal vocational and recovery needs. Participants will benefit, at their own pace, from start to finish with in-person and online job readiness trainings, instructor-led seminars, workshops, trade-specific online academy classes, and finally job placement. Job Launch graduates can expect a newfound purpose and meaning, not only in employment but also in becoming an active member of Safe Harbor's recovery community with immediate in-house access to a variety of peer recovery support groups.[216]

The program is a one-stop shop for jobseekers in any stage of addiction recovery. Employment specialists work closely with participants to:

- Create an individualized program to support their recovery and employment goals.

- Find solutions to overcome obstacles in their employment path.

- Connect participants to other basic needs such as housing, food, childcare, transportation, and healthcare resources as needed.

- Provide one-on-one career exploration, resume development, mock interviews, job application assistance, and job placement.

- Pursue higher education if desired.

Following job placement, the employment specialists continue to work with participants by offering peer-to-peer recovery support services and free access to Safe Harbor computer equipment and business services such as internet access, faxing, copying, scanning, and more.

Spotlight: Working Fields

Working Fields (www.workingfields.com) is a mission-driven staffing agency headquartered in South Burlington, Vermont, with offices in St. Albans, Vermont; Greenfield, Massachusetts; Portsmouth, New Hampshire; and Auburn, Maine. Working Fields participants are in recovery and typically have a criminal record. Founded in 2016 by Mickey Wiles, former CFO for Ben & Jerry's, the agency works with participants by providing job opportunities and peer coaching. They also work hand-in-hand with employers to help them recruit skilled workers looking for a second chance, recognizing that there is an untapped talent pool of people in recovery and with a criminal history.

In addition to job placement services, Working Fields offers two programs:[217]

1. **Peer Coaching:** Peer coaches are trained in strengths-based skills like motivational interviewing, are experts on local resources, and have their own lived experience. They help individuals achieve goals and build stability. One job-seeker said: "My coach encouraged me during a very difficult time in my life and treated me with respect and without judgment."

2. **Return to Work:** The Return to Work program helps businesses provide a *rapid response plan* for employees struggling with substance use, excessive absenteeism, or any other challenge. The program helps businesses decrease costs by retaining skilled employees and connecting struggling employees with trained support.

For employers, Working Fields operates much like other staffing agencies with the added benefits of retention support and expertise in hiring from a diverse population. Businesses identify a role they need to fill on a temporary or temp-to-permanent basis. Working Fields finds, prescreens, and submits a candidate to a business who would be a good fit, saving the business recruitment costs and time. The business has the final say about who to hire.

Working Fields CEO Chelsea Bardot Lewis explains the differentiation of their approach as a placement agency. "Step one is the assessment that we're doing on behalf of the client, the employer. The employer, for example, 'Joe's Auto Shop,' is never going to ask, how's your recovery going? What's your housing situation? What's your relationship status? Those are all the things that we know impact how well someone is going to do at work. But it's not something that the employer is probably going to ask, or perhaps shouldn't. So we do this deep dive with the job seeker on the assessment. We really get to know our client employers. Not just the skill sets, the qualifications, or the required education. We really get to know the culture. We always say retention starts with recruitment.

"We're a retention-focused agency. That starts with where we're recruiting people from, which is from these social service agencies where job seekers are getting additional support. It goes into the assessment that we do, the matchmaking that we do, to make sure that we're getting them the right placement.

"And then, of course, the coaching. So the Human Resource teams love the coaching program, because right now, HR has been stressed, to say the least. Since Covid, they are having employees walk into their office all the time saying, 'I'm losing my apartment, my car broke down.' 'I can't find childcare for my kid; my girlfriend kicked me out.' These are all the things that this one person in HR is dealing with for all the business' frontline workers. Now we at Working Fields can say, 'Listen, this is the job of the coach.' The coach is going to be handling all of that stuff."[218]

What if an employee fails a drug screen? What if they experience a reoccurrence of their substance-use disorder and need to return to treatment?

"Employers do this random drug screening, and then they get the results back, and then they're shocked at the people who are great workers, who come back with something on a drug screen. Because of company policy, the employer has to take an action, because that's their policy. However, the company doesn't want to lose them. Through Return to Work Agreements, a business can adhere to company policy, which is intended to ensure a safe working environment for *all* employees, while simultaneously being compassionate to that worker."

New Hampshire Recovery Friendly Workplace

What is a Recovery Friendly Workplace? The National Recovery Friendly Workplace Institute defines an RFW as "a place of work in which the employer, in collaboration with employees, establishes, maintains, and continually enhances policies, practices, and a culture and work environment that are supportive of current and prospective employees in recovery from, or otherwise affected by, substance use disorders."[219] RFWs adopt policies and practices that:

- Expand employment opportunities for people in or seeking recovery.
- Facilitate help-seeking among employees with substance use disorder (SUD).
- Ensure access to needed services, including treatment, recovery support, and mutual aid.

- Inform employees in recovery that they may have the right to reasonable accommodations and other protections that can help them keep their jobs.

- Reduce the risk of substance use and SUD, including through education and steps to prevent injury in the workplace.

- Educate all levels of the organization on SUD, addiction, and recovery, working to reduce stigma and misunderstanding, including by facilitating open discussion on the topic.

- Ensure that prospective and current employees understand that the workplace is recovery-ready and are familiar with relevant policies and resources.

What began as a New Hampshire statewide initiative in 2018 under the leadership of Governor Chris Sununu has since expanded into a nationwide system with tools, best practices, and technical assistance provided by the National Recovery Friendly Workplace Institute. According to Samantha Lewandowski, senior director of the New Hampshire Recovery Friendly Workplace program, "It all started in March 2018 when the governor, as a former CEO of a New Hampshire ski resort, recalled how his employees were impacted by addiction. Not knowing how to address it at first, his business had to figure it out from scratch. And then when they did have it more figured out, they realized there weren't as many systems in place to kind of refer people to. So then when he became governor he got the Recovery Friendly Workplace program started. Today there are over 380 workplaces participating in the initiative, representing over 95,000 employees."[220]

Jeanne Venuti, New Hampshire RFW director of workforce development, explains how the New Hampshire RFW designation process works. "We designed the process to be simple for businesses. The checklist is one page long, and it starts with a business submitting a letter of interest on our website. It should take less than two minutes to do. It's then going to ping the governor's office as well as us, at which point they will be assigned a recovery friendly advisor who will conduct their orientation with them. The orientation gives them an overview, and takes the business through the checklist, talks about the requirements of the program and how to maintain your designation. The business is asked to provide a declaration to their employees explaining why they decided to become a recovery friendly workplace. Once they submit the declaration to us, we notify the governor's office, and they receive their official designation."[221]

The New Hampshire RFW program became so successful that other states began to reach out to then-director Shannon Swett and the New Hampshire team for help. Lewandowski recalls, "It started snowballing to the point where people from other states were reaching out every single day. And so I thought, well, this is boring for people to keep hearing from just me, so what if we form this community of practice? At the time,

I had around eighty people on my email list and so I set it up. And the attendance was amazing. I have never seen a group who is so committed to showing up. By the time the community of practice transitioned to the national RFW program we had over thirty states represented with over two hundred people on distribution. We got the National Recovery Friendly Workplace Institute launched, and Eliza Zarka, who used to be part of the New Hampshire team on the state side, has taken on the role of the director at the National RFW Institute."

Eliza Zarka is director of state engagement for the institute, and previously worked for the New Hampshire governor's office as an addiction and behavioral health coordinator. She said, "Having a front-row seat to witness the growth of the Recovery Friendly Workplace initiative that was born in a small state like New Hampshire into what is now a truly national movement has been the honor of a lifetime. Becoming a Recovery Friendly Workplace, whether designated by a state-level program or certified by the National Institute, makes good business sense, as you are taking care of people and profit. Accessing quality treatment requires access to quality insurance, and insurance is oftentimes tied to employment, and our places of employment are where we all spend a great deal of time, so, teaching workplaces about substance use and recovery is a natural fit for the culture of this country. Bringing resources and education to where people are, at work, is a significant piece of the puzzle that had been missing, but now companies of any size in any place can take part in this workforce-changing movement."[222]

Maine Recovery Friendly Workplace Program

In 2022, Pinetree Institute was awarded a two-year grant to implement the Recovery Friendly Workplace in the state of Maine. In partnership with the Portland Recovery Community Center, Pinetree Institute developed a program that featured two statewide resources, an RFW Business Advisor to conduct orientation and guide businesses through the RFW certification process, and an RFW Recovery Advisor to conduct training and offer peer recovery support for RFWs.

As of this writing, the Maine RFW program has designated nearly sixty businesses as Recovery Friendly Workplaces with several more in the pipeline. Notably among the Maine RFWs are the University of Maine Augusta and York County Community College. At this time, these educational institutions are the first of their kind in the United States.

The program offers Maine RFWs a structured but flexible engagement model that is customized for the business, connection to statewide and local recovery resources, provides tools and technical assistance, peer support for employees and loved ones, and free training.

Maine Statewide RFW Business Advisor Brittany Reichmann said, "According to national data, over 70 percent of adults with a substance use disorder are employed. We spend more time with our co-workers typically than we do our own families. The workplace can be one of the most influential places to support individuals. It isn't just about people in recovery, or people struggling with substance use issues, it's also about the person who shows up to work every day whose life is in chaos because someone they love is using drugs or alcohol. This is a wellness initiative, it's about supporting people, however it is that they are affected—bottom line."[223]

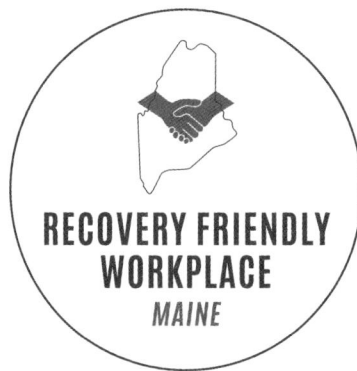

Figure 11: Maine Recovery Friendly Workplace Logo.

Designation: The process of becoming a Maine RFW begins with a business submitting a letter of interest (LOI) to the Maine RFW program office managed by Pinetree Institute. Once the business attends an RFW orientation and declares in writing to their employees their commitment to become an RFW, the business is officially designated as a Maine RFW. At that point, the business is sent a congratulatory letter and RFW welcome kit. The kit includes the Maine RFW official logo images, a logo usage guideline, menu of available trainings, contact information, and a copy of the RFW checklist regarding next steps.

Training: The first four modules are required within the first year of designation. Sessions are approximately one hour long and available in person or virtually.

1. Substance Use Disorder 101

    a. General information including prevalence data and clinical criteria

    b. ACEs, protective factors, and warning signs explained

    c. Discussion around stigma and person-centered language

    d. Actionable tips for coworkers and loved ones to address developing SUDs

2. Opioid Overdose Response

   a. What is naloxone?

   b. Discuss the signs of an opioid-related emergency

   c. Review strategies, protocols, and best practices to address overdose

   d. Create a workplace environment that prioritizes safety and well-being

3. Recovery 101

   a. Principles and pathways to recovery and systems of care that include employers

   b. Explanation of common principles of successful recovery and personal, social, and community-based elements that support individual recovery

   c. Exploration of how employers may fit into the ecosystem of recovery support.

   d. Employee self-care, mental health, and wellness

4. Growing Your Recovery Friendly Workplace

   a. Discuss existing protocols for addressing substance use

   b. Being a trauma-informed workplace

   c. Diversity, equity, inclusion, and fair chance hiring practices

   d. How can businesses put new learning into sustainable action?

Access to Services

Across the entire recovery-oriented system of care, lack of access to services, whether transportation or technology, is a major barrier. For transportation this could be lack of owning a car, not having a valid or active driver's license, or not having reliable public transportation. From a technology perspective, this could be lack of Wi-Fi or cellular service, lack of a computer or phone, or technology illiteracy.

Lack of access prevents individuals and families from getting to a meeting, an appointment, or a visit to a recovery community organization. In the dawning age of teleservices, not having a phone, computer, data plan or Wi-Fi access prevents folks from accessing these virtual services. This also can result in a person being isolated from their family or their recovery supports.

Many recovery community organizations offer bus passes, Uber or Lyft fares, or in some areas, actual rides for people. Some communities, such as the Greater Portsmouth Recovery Coalition and Strafford County Public Health Network, have offered free smartphones with prepaid data plans.

Re-entry Services

The negative health implications of incarceration disproportionately impact individuals living with mental health and substance use disorder. Jail and prison settings often involve risk of assault, isolation, coercion, and intimidation.[224, 225] Individuals living with co-occurring mental health and substance use disorders are more likely to experience victimization or exploitation while in prison, making their experience behind bars worse.[226]

Individuals living with mental health and substance use disorders who reenter the community following incarceration often encounter significant barriers to treatment, housing, meaningful employment, and other services. Appropriate reentry services for the formerly incarcerated can reduce risk for recurrence and recidivism as well as risk of overdose, self-harm, or risky behavior leading to reincarceration.

Re-entry planning helps prepare inmates to achieve long-term post-release success. From the perspective of the inmate preparing for release, significant anxiety emerges about issues the rest of us may take for granted. For example, where will I live? Can I find a job? What about my record? Can I reunite with my family? Where do I go to get recovery support?[227]

A recovery ready community is set up to provide a transition from prerelease to re-entry into the community, addressing all of these needs for the justice involved.

Example: Maine Reentry Network (MERN)

Bruce Noddin seems to show up everywhere I happen to be in my travels around the state of Maine. Recovery Day celebrations in Auburn, the Governor's Opioid Summit in Portland, a community coalition kick-off in Sanford, a Recovery Friendly Workplace event in Augusta. As the executive director and founder of the Maine Reentry Network (MERN), Noddin has good reason to network across the state. He said, "I started doing a jail ministry at the Androscoggin County Jail, and we were seeing the same guys coming back every week, it was every Thursday that we were there, and I was seeing these poor guys coming back week after week, month after month, year after year. And we were asking the question, you know, what? What are we doing for these folks when they leave?"[228]

"What did you learn by asking around?" I asked him.

"The answer to that question of what we are doing for these folks when they leave incarceration was nothing," he said. "Just release people, let them go. So we started to have meetings. First, Catholic Charities gave us an office in Auburn, and we noticed that people were driving from an hour and a half to two hours away to talk about reentry, which blew my mind. And we were trying to get as many disparate organizations that could have a part in somebody's reentry recovery to attend."

How did it evolve?

"We started out with five guys, and then the next month, they were twelve, the next month they were over twenty, the next month we had to move across the street to the church because we ran out of space. And then we realized that we really needed to take the show on the road. So we started having monthly meetings in Augusta, Bangor, Midcoast, eventually up in Aroostook County, western Maine. We met in the county jails, the county sheriffs' offices, within the community itself. So most of the meetings were community meetings."

What were the meetings like within the jails? How did the inmates react?

"We had a number of men who had been in prison before, and one gentleman in particular, Peter Lehman, who is part of the Maine Prisoner Advocacy Coalition," Noddin said. "Peter was a liaison to our meetings from the coalition. He and I started going in together, and I noticed, because I first started going in by myself, and I've never been in prison or jail, so when Peter came and introduced himself as having spent six years at Maine State Prison, everything changed. The body language of the group changed. Trust was instantly established. That peer relationship thing again, it all comes down to lived experience. And if somebody hasn't been through what you've been through, then it's hard to really trust them. So that's when we discovered that going together in pairs was a much better approach as each one of us was seeing something different in the conversations. And most of what we were doing was listening. We were listening for what direction that person wanted to go in, and then from the piles of resources that we'd established all over the state we could talk about some of the resources that were available to them. And then COVID hit. COVID made us a more effective, better organization, because we carried that Zoom meeting approach to today."

What are the services that MERN provides?

"We provide peer reentry/recovery support for people that are in Maine's state prisons, county jails, and in federal prisons if requested," Noddin said. "We have a memorandum of understanding with the Department of Corrections whereas the reentry process needs to start at a minimum of nine months prior to release. So we start doing these Zoom meetings, and then we start to introduce the resources to inmates preparing for reentry. We invite workforce development folks, we invite people that own recovery residences, recovery coaches, peer support from a recovery community center, and we invite family members if that's important to the person. We're really following their lead, but we're giving them suggestions about what's available."

Today, MERN meets by Zoom every Tuesday for ninety minutes and is attended by between fifty and as many as eighty prisoners in the re-entry program, partners, providers, volunteers, and community-based organizations that provide services to prisoners upon re-entry.

CHAPTER 16

OTHER IMPORTANT TOPICS

Rural Communities

Rural communities are often separated by social services and medical care by time and distance. Although the majority of America's population is concentrated in urban and suburban settings, the vast majority of our country is considered rural. According to the US Census Bureau, urban areas make up only 3 percent of the land area of the US but are home to more than 80 percent of the population. On the other hand, 97 percent of the US land area is considered rural, but only 19.3 percent (about sixty million people) live in rural settings.[229]

A 2022 study conducted by the University of Vermont Center on Rural Addiction (CORA) cited the following barriers to treating patients for Opioid Use Disorders (OUD) in the state of Maine:

- Rural practitioners cite lack of time, transportation, housing, and "other supports" as the top barriers facing their patients receiving treatment for OUD.

- Rural practitioners also identify time and staffing constraints, and fear of medication diversion, as their own barriers for treating patients with OUD.

- Rural community stakeholders cited transportation, housing, lack of care coordination, and lack of capacity to treat patients for OUD within their communities.[230]

In a separate study among family members and people in treatment in rural Vermont, the following themes emerged:[231]

- Lack of transportation, insurance, stable housing, and financial stability were identified as barriers to initiating and maintaining treatment engagement.

- Clinic settings were described as often having inflexible policies and treatment environments not conducive to patient-centered care.

- Continuity of care was identified as vital for high quality treatment (e.g., meeting regularly with the same health provider).

- Stigma associated with OUD was perceived to increase the need for compassionate, patient-centered care.

- Positive social connections were identified as a need, particularly with peers who share common goals.

- Some people in treatment and family members viewed Medications for Opioid Use Disorder (MOUD) as a continuing tie to opioid dependence.

Maine's Department of Health and Human Services does a great job of outreach through technology. At the 2024 Maine Governor's Opioid Summit in Lewiston, I picked up a rack card that listed strategies for reducing harm from alcohol use and opioid use. What struck me with the rack card and most of the other literature I collected that day was that QR codes were used to connect people to services offered by the agency handing out the literature. Telehealth and teleservices are vital to provide access to people who may not have reliable transportation, yet live miles away from these services.

Not everyone in rural communities have access to a phone, computer, or internet connectivity. In these communities, in-home services such as that offered by organizations such as Aware Recovery Care provide an opportunity for those in remote locations to access service.

Safe supplies, life-saving naloxone, and other physical harm reduction supplies cannot be delivered via technology. Brick and mortar or mobile services are essential for rural communities, not just in Maine, but across the US. Chapter 14 provides an example of teleservices and in particular, Better Life Partners, an agency whose business model is specifically intended to reach rural populations.

Addressing NIMBYism

Most of us know that the acronym NIMBY is shorthand for "Not In My Backyard" and often represents opposition to a development or entity due to fear of loss of property value. Examples include the opening of an adult bookstore or casino in a section of a town that requires approvals of variances, usually to the opposition of neighbors.

In the recovery space, opening a recovery community organization or a recovery home is often met with opposition for similar reasons. Neighbors sometimes oppose such entities due to concerns about "drug addicts selling dope" in the neighborhood or other such irrational fears, often ignoring evidence to the contrary.

Sometimes opposition can perpetuate stigmatizing tropes about people in recovery. Town meetings, public hearings and zoning board meetings can attract both proponents and opponents of recovery-related development projects. Transparent proposals, open and respectful communication, and "meeting the opposition where they are at" approaches can provide opportunities to lower the temperature and to educate the community on the facts about addiction, recovery, and re-entry.

The Fletcher Group has developed a guide to handling NIMBYism in the community, in this case for recovery housing, which is a methodology based on best practices, and a checklist "for an effective, proactive response."[232]

1. **Prepare Early:** Work slowly and carefully, especially at the beginning, building momentum over time.

2. **Address Legitimate Concerns:** Respond earnestly to all concerns.

3. **Recruit Allies:** Local knowledge is the key to success, so honor and defer to local stakeholders.

4. **Start Now:** Begin as soon as possible to identify and bring onboard community leaders who can mobilize support.

5. **Local Leadership:** Recruit well-known and trusted leaders to be the face of the project.

6. **Organize:** Enlist allies to form a NIMBY Committee.

7. **Anticipate:** Anticipate barriers and prepare for them.

8. **Showcase Success:** Document outcomes with facts and data including video and in-person testimonials.

9. **Stress Public Safety:** Counter concerns of nefarious behavior, violence, and crime by showing how the facility will be the least likely place to find such things.

10. **Take the High Road:** Treat detractors with respect.

11. **Communicate:** Identify and repeat key messages through a wide range of media.

12. **Media Relations:** Seek opportunities to write articles based on interviews with people in recovery.

Example: SOS Recovery Community Organization— Hampton, New Hampshire

In 2019, SOS Recovery Community Organization, with locations in Dover and Rochester, New Hampshire, opened its third location, on Route 1 / Lafayette Road in Hampton. SOS provides a variety of peer recovery supports including meetings, peer recovery support services such as recovery coaching and telephone recovery supports, crisis navigation and a variety of activities such as yoga, art in recovery, music in recovery, and social activities.

The opening was significant as the organization, led by Executive Director John Burns, was anything but a sure thing. SOS held a series of information sessions over the early spring at the Hampton Police Department and presented the proposal to the board of selectmen. I attended each of these sessions in support of the program along with several other community and state officials who supported SOS's expansion.

Following a presentation by Burns at the initial information session, a few concerned parents and one of the five Hampton selectmen raised concerns about the location, its potential proximity to schools, and the participants who would be visiting the center. It should be noted that a location had not been selected.

Despite the fact that the concerns were based largely on a lack of understanding of facts and statistics, Burns listened carefully and acknowledged the concerns raised by these attendees. Supporters of the program spoke about the value to the community since at that time we were seeing a surge in overdoses in the area. John provided links to reference materials and handed out some flyers that helped to explain what the center does and the benefits to the community. Again, he leaned into the conversation without dismissing the concerns of the opposition.

At the second meeting, some of those who were concerned came to voice their support after doing a bit of homework on their own. At the town selectmen meeting, the proposal was approved by a majority vote and the center opened several months later.

TIP: When facing NIMBYism in your efforts to build recovery capacity, lean in to your opposition's concerns and meet them where they are at. It is easier to push a wheelbarrow on level ground.

SECTION 4

THE GREATER PORTSMOUTH RECOVERY COALITION—A CASE STUDY

BACKGROUND

The Greater Portsmouth Recovery Coalition was anything but that in the early days of its formation. In 2018, there was no blueprint for building a recovery ready community. There were no templates or best practices to draw on for a fast start. Like many other communities across New Hampshire and indeed, the rest of the country, community leaders were struggling to stem the tide against fatal overdoses from opioids. The community did what it had to do and with the resources immediately available to care for its own.

Consider that time period was pre-COVID. We did not yet have millions of dollars flowing into states' attorneys general offices from pharmaceutical and Sackler settlements. Widespread acceptance of recovery housing, medication-assisted treatment (MAT), and harm reduction had not yet occurred. Families and communities were desperate for solutions.

The city of Portsmouth, New Hampshire, is a port city on the southern shore of the Piscataqua River and is the northernmost community on New Hampshire's modest thirteen-mile coast. In the nearly forty years that we have lived on what is known as the Seacoast of New Hampshire, Portsmouth has transformed from a lower- to middle-class community with a charming downtown area comprised of shops, restaurants, and professional offices to one of the most desirable and expensive places to live in New England.

Portsmouth is an incorporated city with an elected city council and hired city manager. The mayor of Portsmouth emerges as the councilor receiving the most votes in a two-year election cycle. The median family income in Portsmouth has soared from $59,630 in 2000[233] to $124,789 in 2024. [234]

As evidence of this economic growth, my wife and I purchased a new six-room two-story home with a single-stall attached garage that was situated on a tiny one-quarter acre lot for $99,500 in 1985. We sold that home in 1991 for around $150,000. Zillow values that home today at $802,100.[235] Regardless of the socioeconomic status of Portsmouth and the surrounding Seacoast towns, the New Hampshire opioid epidemic is painfully present.

Since 2016, New Hampshire has had the ignominious reputation of having one of the highest per capita fatal overdose rates in the country with more than three times the national average.[236] A 2017 *US News & World Report* article cited New Hampshire as ground zero in the United States for the opioid crisis due to its "lack of funding for treatment, its rural context, and high (opiate) prescription rates."[237] The cities of Manchester,

Nashua, Rochester, and Dover have been hit especially hard with some of the highest per capita overdose deaths in the country. Other New Hampshire communities such as Laconia, Keene, Concord, and Berlin were not far behind.[238] Portsmouth, a Seacoast city of approximately twenty-two thousand citizens and one of the wealthiest communities in the state, has not been immune. Between 2016 and 2024, the city of Portsmouth has averaged five fatal overdoses per year.

In 2023, the University of New Hampshire Institute for Health Policy and Practice and the Foundation for Seacoast Health funded the *Seacoast-Area Health Assessments Review* to determine healthcare priorities for the region. The study consolidated the independent community health assessments conducted by Exeter Hospital (New Hampshire), Seacoast Public Health Network (New Hampshire), Wentworth-Douglass Hospital (New Hampshire), York Hospital (Maine), York County (Maine), and York County Community Action Program. Below is a summary of the consolidated findings. In aggregate, respondents included educators, providers, law enforcement, first responders, hospitals, and the public. As you can see, the categories of Mental and Behavioral Health and SUD are the only common priority areas across all six studies.[239]

Priority Areas	Exeter Hospital CHNA	Seacoast Public Health Network CHIP	York Hospital CHNA	York County, Maine Shared CHNA	York County Community Action Corp. CNA	Wentworth-Douglass Hosptial CHNA
Access to Care	✓		✓	✓	✓	✓
Physical Health		✓				✓
Mental and Behavioral Health	✓	✓	✓	✓	✓	✓
Substance Use	✓	✓	✓	✓	✓	✓
Older Adults and Other Underserved Populations	✓	✓			✓	✓
Social Determinants of Health						
Economic Stability	✓			✓	✓	✓
Education	✓			✓	✓	✓
Food Security	✓			✓		✓
Housing	✓			✓	✓	✓
Transportation	✓			✓	✓	✓
Broadband Access				✓		
Social and Community Context	✓			✓	✓	

Table 2: Healthcare Priorities for Eastern New Hampshire and Southern Maine.

This Greater Portsmouth Recovery Coalition might be the most comprehensive example of building a community coalition to address SUD in the country when considering the multiphase, five-year program that delivered tangible outcomes. The coalition expanded in membership and scope despite occurring over three city elections, COVID-19, and multiple grant cycles. The coalition is still in operation to this day.

This case study documents the entire lifecycle of the Greater Portsmouth Recovery Coalition across Assessment, Capacity, Planning, Implementation, Evaluation, and Sustainability phases as outlined earlier in the SAMHSA Strategic Prevention Framework. It bears repeating that we built and sustained this coalition without having this framework or any other blueprint to guide us. Where appropriate, we highlight tips and other suggestions based on our learning.

Evolution of the Greater Portsmouth Recovery Coalition

- **2018:** Conversations with community leaders and interested groups.

- **2019:** Portsmouth community breakout group at Pinetree Resilience Conference, discussion of collaboration options.

- **2019:** Launch of Portsmouth Coordinated Response to SUD, identification of top priority needs for focus.

- **2020–2021:** Initial phases of Coordinated Response with task forces focusing on key priority areas and significant accomplishments.

- **2022–2023:** Establishment of Greater Portsmouth Recovery Coalition, maintaining focus on initial priorities, and expanding to address emerging issues. Recognize greater Portsmouth as a Recovery Ready Community.

- **2023–2024:** Measuring Outcomes.

Timeline of the Greater Portsmouth Recovery Coalition

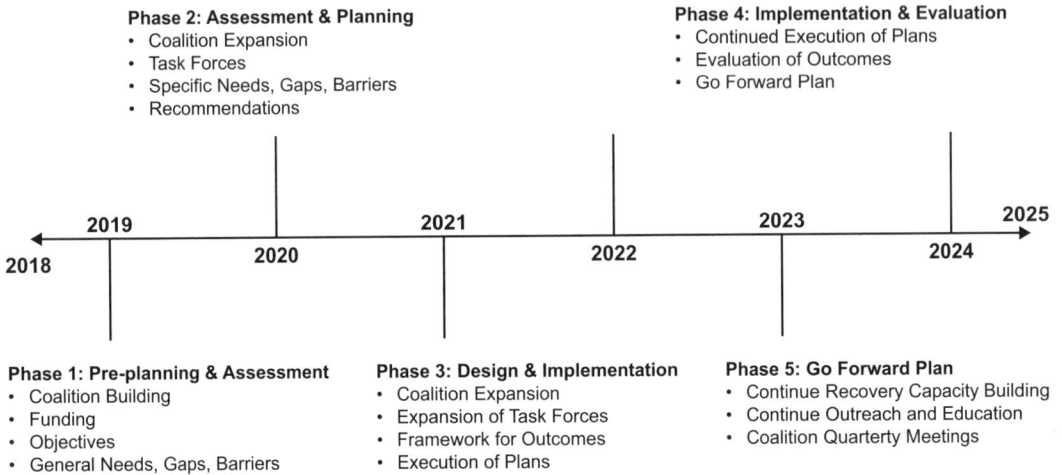

Phase 2: Assessment & Planning
- Coalition Expansion
- Task Forces
- Specific Needs, Gaps, Barriers
- Recommendations

Phase 4: Implementation & Evaluation
- Continued Execution of Plans
- Evaluation of Outcomes
- Go Forward Plan

2018 — 2019 — 2020 — 2021 — 2022 — 2023 — 2024 — 2025

Phase 1: Pre-planning & Assessment
- Coalition Building
- Funding
- Objectives
- General Needs, Gaps, Barriers

Phase 3: Design & Implementation
- Coalition Expansion
- Expansion of Task Forces
- Framework for Outcomes
- Execution of Plans

Phase 5: Go Forward Plan
- Continue Recovery Capacity Building
- Continue Outreach and Education
- Coalition Quarterly Meetings

Figure 12: Greater Portsmouth Recovery Coalition Timeline.

The Community Recovery Landscape (2018)

Before the formation of the coalition, there were organizations in the region that provided direct SUD services:

- **The Doorway (New Hampshire):** The Doorway was founded in February 2019 under the Sununu administration and provides single points of entry for people seeking help for SUD. The nine regional Doorways are located such that help is available an hour or less away and provides 24/7 access by dialing 2-1-1. The Doorway connects participants to the appropriate level of services and level of care that includes screening, evaluation, treatment (today including MAT), prevention (naloxone), and peer recovery support services.[240]

- **Seacoast Mental Health Center:** Seacoast Mental Health Center provides evidence-based mental health services to the residents of the eastern half of Rockingham County, with locations in Portsmouth and Exeter, New Hampshire.

- **Safe Harbor Recovery Center:** Safe Harbor Recovery is a recovery community organization (RCO) founded in 2015. Safe Harbor, which operates under the nonprofit organization Granite Pathways, provides support to individuals seeking recovery or those who want to be part of the recovery community. Safe Harbor at the time of its founding was just the second RCO in the state of New Hampshire.

- **SOS Recovery Community Organization:** A peer-driven recovery community organization with locations in Dover, Rochester, and Hampton, New Hampshire. The Hampton location has since been relocated to Exeter.

- **Portsmouth Regional Hospital:** The Behavioral Health Unit offers inpatient admission, involuntary emergency admission, an outpatient partial hospital program, 24/7 crisis and referral hotline, and community programs.

- **Addiction Recovery Services:** ARSNH provides evidence-based intensive outpatient (IOP), group therapy, family education, and medication management, with a focus on the co-occurring mental health symptoms accompanying addiction.

- **Dozens of LADC/Alcohol & Drug Counselors**

In 2018 there was no widespread access to medication-assisted treatment (MAT) or harm reduction services in the greater Portsmouth community. There were no recovery homes within Rockingham County. There were no re-entry services for individuals re-entering the community upon release from the Rockingham or nearby Strafford County jails. And there were few if any services to assist families impacted by recovery. What we did have was a motivated and well-connected set of concerned officials, organizations, and volunteers who wanted to address the growing need for addiction prevention, treatment, and recovery services in the community. They came together in 2019.

Creating the Coalition (2019)

Some of the most hopeful responses to the SUD challenge have come from communities that have taken a comprehensive, trauma-informed approach to care. Communities began to recognize that many of the challenges in addiction and co-occurring mental health issues have their roots in childhood adversity and trauma and cannot be effectively addressed unless the root causes are acknowledged.

In May 2019, then State Senator Martha Fuller Clark gathered a small group of leaders from Portsmouth to discuss the state's epidemic, the impact, and ways to mitigate the issue locally. In New Hampshire, the death rate had climbed close to four hundred persons per year in 2017 and 2018; the state had one of the highest per capita rates of overdose deaths in the nation. The ad hoc committee recognized that not only was this a personal and community tragedy, but it was also placing increasing demands on already strained community resources. Additionally, there was substantial economic and social impact.

New Hampshire Superior Court Chief Justice Tina Nadeau was another early participant on the initial committee. "I was excited that there was a grassroots effort to come up with some concrete ideas to deal with the opioid epidemic. I'm so used to government being part of groups and committees that study issues and write reports, all of which are important. But this group was so active and so engaged at a grassroots level that it inspired me to be involved. I spent my career developing and increasing the access to drug courts in our superior court system. So it was a perfect marriage of two ideas whereby I felt comfortable being involved."[241]

Dr. Larry McCullough, executive director at Pinetree Institute, recalls the series of events that led to this initial gathering. "Pinetree Institute had just hosted our first Resilience Conference, which was held in Portsmouth and featured Dr. Robert Anda and Laura Porter, co-founders of ACE Interface, LLC. Here we had a group of people from Portsmouth sitting around in a circle, saying, 'How would understanding ACEs impact what we would do in our community?' So we started talking about the issues."[242]

McCullough continued, "We asked ourselves, 'Wouldn't we need representatives from all the different organizations to work together? Wouldn't we need to figure out the needs across the community?' And that was really the birth of this idea of a community coalition to address recovery."

During that meeting conversations among participants from many organizations across the community and with personnel from Pinetree Institute of Eliot, Maine, and Portsmouth, New Hampshire, suggested that engaging in a formal planning process would be helpful in creating a coordinated plan for action. This planning process would look at the requirements for coordination across the various agencies and sectors that provide services and are impacted by the substance use disorder crisis. The discussions would also specifically address requirements across the full range of the continuum of care: prevention treatment and recovery support.

Pinetree Institute was asked to provide a facilitator to work with this inaugural steering committee and recruited a larger group of stakeholders to determine the present level of need and to identify gaps and overlaps. This request led to a facilitated session to understand the needs of each sector of the community and help to create a plan for coordinated action.

COVID-19

On March 11, 2020, the World Health Organization (WHO) declared COVID-19 a pandemic. The impact to the coalition was significant as many members of the steering committee and task forces were called on to serve the community during this crisis. During the pandemic, nearly all indicators—overdose deaths, Narcan administrations by EMS workers, SUD related hospital admissions—declined significantly.

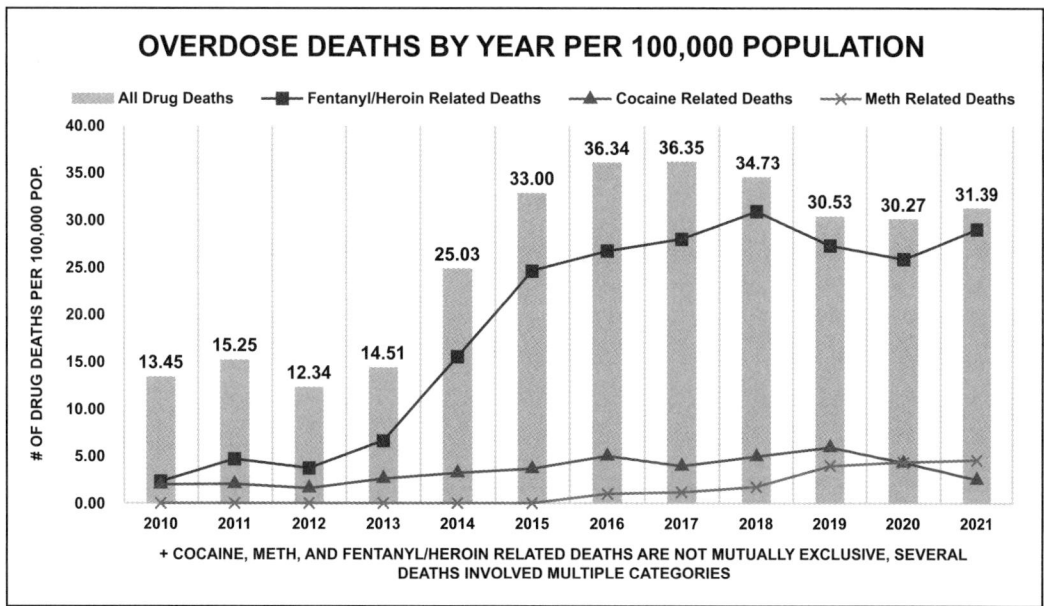

OVERDOSE DEATHS BY YEAR PER 100,000 POPULATION

Figure 13: NH Overdose Deaths By Year Per 100,000 Population.[243] (NHDHHS)

Undaunted by the pandemic, the coalition marched forward with convenings of the steering committee and task forces conducted through Zoom video conferences.

> **TIP:** The coalition should be prepared to adapt when unforeseen factors arise.

Phase 1: Pre-Planning (2019)

Cliff Lazenby was the assistant mayor of Portsmouth in 2019 and became interested in the movement to address substance use after seeing the local film *The Heroin Effect* a few years prior. Lazenby has since retired from the city council and now works in the hospitality industry. Lazenby recalls, "The type of people we brought together were motivated to talk to other people about what we can do by bringing like-minded people together, but in a coordinated fashion. I remember we were in a conference room at City Hall, and State Senator Fuller Clark had spoken about the topic with then-Mayor Jack Blalock. We also had a fire chief, the police chief, Seacoast Mental Health, and the hospital. We had all these people in the room and listening to what people are doing or what they would like to do about SUD in the community. And we thought, 'This would be better if we coordinated this work.' But every single person there had their own job to do. Which is where Pinetree Institute stepped in, as here was an organization that had experience working with groups of people in a coordinated way.

"Early on we got some great help from a financial standpoint, to just help pay for that coordination time. So the Portsmouth Rotary and the city of Portsmouth put some initial money up that first time around to help pay for the services of Pinetree Institute and to have Larry work with the rest of us."[244]

Setting Objectives of the Planning Process

The steering committee of the Greater Portsmouth Recovery Coalition sought to establish a baseline of community assets and capabilities. The exercise allowed the committee to set priorities and expand the coalition with these priorities in mind.

- Create an initial analysis of current needs and existing services as well as known service gaps.
- Engage key stakeholders and decision makers in a dialogue about areas for potential coordination.
- Research and provide information on successful strategies to address the substance use crisis in other parts of the US, particularly trauma-informed strategies that provide a base for cross-sector collaboration.
- Recommend steps for future action including service gaps and overlaps to address, plans for communitywide dialogue and education, and mechanisms to ensure coordination can be built into ongoing operating plans.

TIP: Research best practices and assess current capacity against these best practices.

With this set of initial objectives defined, the steering committee set in motion the next steps to expand the coalition in a coordinated and focused manner. The committee sought to recruit stakeholders that aligned with the coalition objectives.

Proposed Planning Steps

- Cooperate with members of the steering committee representing ten to twelve key agencies and organizations and identify other stakeholders to be included in the planning process.
- Create an initial analysis of current needs and status of services including meetings with key service providers, stakeholders and client groups, and review of existing

data to create a "snapshot" of current state. (Note: this is not a comprehensive needs analysis but a rapid collection and organization of existing data from important stakeholder groups.)

- Meet with steering committee to review current status and identify participants to be included in coordination discussions.

- Hold discussions with individuals and groups identified by the steering committee. Some conversations would be one-on-one, some would be small groups.

- Create a draft plan and recommendations. Based on the broader stakeholder discussions, identify key themes, findings, and recommendations for next steps.

- Conduct review meeting with steering committee to approve recommendations and agree on next steps.

It was at this time that the coalition formally identified itself as the Portsmouth Coordinated Response to Substance Use Disorder.

TIP: Don't overthink this initial needs assessment at this early phase. At this stage, the coalition is setting priorities for the group to move forward with the best information available at that time.

Steering Committee Representation

The initial steering committee was comprised of a cross-sector of leaders to address priorities and assess the city's capacity to address SUD. I include this list to emphasize the cross-sector organization representation, but perhaps more significant, the commitment of decision-makers that participated.

- Portsmouth City Council: Assistant Mayor Cliff Lazenby (committee chair)

- New Hampshire State Senate: Martha Fuller Clark, state senator, district 21

- New Hampshire Superior Court: Tina Nadeau, chief justice, New Hampshire Superior Court

- Child Advocacy Center, Rockingham County: Maureen Sullivan, executive director

- Rockingham County Department of Corrections: Stephen Church, superintendent

- Portsmouth Police Department: Robert Merner, chief; Darrin Sargent, lieutenant, investigative division

- Portsmouth Fire Department: Todd Germain, chief

- Portsmouth School Department: Stephen Zadravec, Superintendent; Christine Burke, wellness coordinator
- Portsmouth Economic Development Commission: Alan Gold
- Portsmouth Hospital: Grant Turpin, EMS/outreach director; Stephen Curtis, behavioral health director
- Seacoast Mental Health Center: Jay Couture, executive director; Diane Fontneau, SUD program manager
- Safe Harbor Recovery Center: Heather Blumenfeld, director
- Granite Pathways: Patricia Reed, New Hampshire state director
- HAVEN: Kathy Beebe, executive director; Sarah Shanahan, program director
- Portsmouth Housing Authority: Tammy Joslyn, residential services coordinator
- Chamber Collaborative of Greater Portsmouth: Valerie Rochon, president
- Pinetree Institute: Dr. Larry McCullough, executive director

TIP: Make the most of the availability of the coalition members in this initial stage. The coalition does not need to have 100 percent participation at each meeting to move forward.

From this initial convening of the steering committee, the following priority focus areas were defined. These focus areas would serve as the pivot for the coalition to expand with stakeholders who were working with or connected to these priority areas:

1. Community Education & Training in ACEs
2. Recovery Housing
3. Employment
4. Transportation
5. Case Management and Coordinated Referral

Output of Pre-Planning Process

The Portsmouth Coordinated Response to SUD Steering Committee met four times between July and November 2019. During those meetings, the group discussed the current status of response to substance use, identified major gaps in services, and identified several areas that required additional attention. Below are the recommendations that emerged from the Pre-Planning Phase of the coalition. (It should be noted that this report is written in present tense as reported out in 2019.)

1. **Extend the Coordinated Response Steering Committee** for a period of one year (July 2019 to June 2020) to manage a set of task forces focused on the priority areas identified by the initial steering committee. All members of the initial committee will be invited to extend their service or nominate a representative. Additional members may be invited as determined by the ongoing committee. The ongoing steering committee would be facilitated similarly to the 2019 steering committee and would meet every other month for a total of six meetings to review the work of the task forces and develop recommendations as appropriate.

    • Provide for management and facilitation of the coordination process for a period of one year, support the work of the task forces and draft recommendations for action as they are developed including an interim and final summary report. A budget for professional facilitation and potential funding sources would be detailed in early 2020.

    • In addition to the five specific task forces, the steering committee will work on two areas with impact across all priority areas: identifying sources for funding and resource development and establishing appropriate baseline and ongoing metrics to measure the impact of actions proposed by the task forces. The facilitator and steering committee will ensure that each task force addresses issues of potential funding and identifies ways that success might be measured. They will also encourage each task force to identify best practices being implemented in other communities and assess their relevance for application in Portsmouth.

2. **Create Five Task Forces** to develop recommended actions in five of the priority areas identified by the initial steering committee as follows:

    • **Community Education and Training in ACEs, Trauma-informed Care, and Prevention:** The committee agreed there is a need for more preventive educational programs for families, children, and youth including social-emotional learning and specific substance use understanding that this task force will address. One of the top needs identified is for greater awareness and training on the topic of adverse childhood experiences (ACEs) and trauma-informed care both for the professional service community and for the general public. Several initiatives are underway including a Master Training program being developed by Pinetree Institute.

- **Recovery Housing:** Sober housing and transitional housing options are major gaps in the Portsmouth area with currently no sober housing options available within easy reach. The full range of housing needs for individuals in recovery and transition needs considerable attention and no easy solutions are currently identified. This task force will further clarify current gaps and identify priorities for development for near- and long-term solutions.

- **Employment:** Employment after treatment and transition back into the workforce is a major factor for people attempting to manage a successful recovery. There are significant new programs such as New Hampshire Works for Recovery that can assist with this process which are just now getting full attention in the Portsmouth area. This task force will work to ensure that this program and others like it are being fully utilized and identify other areas in which support for employment can be augmented.

- **Transportation:** Transportation was identified as a major gap with very few existing options that can provide support. The underlying issue is one of access, and even where services are available, without affordable transportation options and ways to support transportation needs it is difficult for individuals to take advantage of those services. The transportation task force will examine current options and will primarily be charged with exploring new options for transportation and funding that don't currently exist.

- **Case Management and Coordinated Referral:** Helping individuals in recovery navigate the complex maze of services and eligibility requirements is a significant need that usually falls in the cracks between the service mandates of organizations. The Doorway in Dover, New Hampshire, is one attempt to address this issue, but the director of the Doorway told the steering committee that the Portsmouth area is still greatly underserved. This task force will address the issue of care coordination, which includes approaches to case management, and also explore issues related to shared information, service planning, and access to services.

We did not call this a charter at the time; however, in hindsight, this was the tacit agreement between coalition stakeholders regarding the constitution of the steering committee and our priorities going forward. Funding for this pre-planning phase was provided by the city of Portsmouth, New Hampshire Rotary, and the Foundation for Seacoast Health.

TIP: Be sure to document the output of each and every phase of the coalition lifecycle. Store all digital documents in a secure folder as well as a backup folder in the cloud.

Phase 2: Planning (2020)

In January 2020, I joined Pinetree Institute and took on the role of program director for the coalition.

Now that the coalition was armed with a set of recommendations that were based on thoughtful deliberation from the steering committee, the next phase would involve building committees or task forces to develop detailed plans and recommendations for each of the five priorities of Community Education, Recovery Housing, Employment, Transportation, and Services Coordination.

In addition to the steering committee, which convened quarterly and was comprised of sector leaders across the community, a so-called "Leadership Committee" was also formed for governance of the coalition. The leadership committee ensured the coalition task forces and steering committee advanced forward and the work aligned with the coalition mission and goals. Larry McCullough and Mark Lefebvre from Pinetree Institute, Alan Gold from the city's Economic Development Commission, and Cliff Lazenby, assistant mayor of the city of Portsmouth, served on this committee. The committee convened monthly.

TIP: Establish a coalition leadership committee to ensure the advancement of the coalition remains aligned with coalition mission and goals.

The five task forces were created to advance the priorities proposed by the steering committee in September 2019. Membership of the task forces began with a steering committee member acting as de facto co-chair for each of the five task forces, and the committee reached out through their networks to recruit prospective task force members.

Over the course of the next twelve months, each of the task forces formed their respective teams and set up monthly working meetings. For each task force, the goal was to assess current needs and capabilities, identify gaps and barriers, and lay out a set of recommendations for each of the five priorities brought forward from Phase 1.

Pinetree Institute continued its role as coalition facilitator during Phase 2. The final report would be presented to the steering committee with quarterly reports on task force progress. These recommendations would be presented to the steering committee to consider beyond Phase 2.

The five task forces were:

1. Community Education and Training
2. Housing
3. Employment
4. Access / Connectivity
5. Services Coordination

Following is the final report presented to the steering committee at the end of Phase 2.

1. Community Education and Training in ACEs, Trauma-informed Care, and Prevention

The committee agreed there is a need for more preventive educational programs for families, children, and youth. One of the top needs identified is for greater awareness and training on the topic of adverse childhood experiences (ACEs) and trauma-informed care both for the professional service community and for the general public. Several initiatives are underway including a Master Training program being implemented by Pinetree Institute.

Task Force Members:
Christine Burke, wellness coordinator, Portsmouth Schools
Sarah Shanahan, education & training director, Haven
Maureen Sullivan, executive director, New Hampshire Child Advocacy Center
Larry McCullough, Mark Lefebvre, Pinetree Institute

Objectives:
- Prevent substance use disorder through education and outreach.
- Reduce the stigma of childhood trauma.
- Evaluate existing prevention-oriented training programs within the Portsmouth school system.
- Complete an inventory of existing services.
- Identify organizations for ACEs and other prevention-oriented training.
- Evaluate best practices in other parts of the state.
- Issue report with findings and recommendations.

Needs: The task force determined that the greatest need for education is for those organizations that provide direct services to children, youth, and young adults. These include recreational organizations, afterschool programs, youth sports organizations, teachers, caregivers, clinical providers, and any other group or organization that serve these populations.

Educational curricula include the effect that ACEs have on individual, family, and public health, evidence-based best practices on how to mitigate this impact, and the positive impact of positive childhood experiences (PCEs) to build resilience for individuals, families, and communities.

Results: The task force created a substantial database of organizations and programs that offer services to youth and young adults. This database includes those programs that are statewide, regional, and local to the greater Portsmouth community.

The task force is focused on greater awareness and training to such organizations, particularly around trauma as a root cause of mental and behavioral health issues. Training and education initiatives that are underway focus on the topic of ACEs, PCEs, and related trauma-informed care, and are designed both for the professional service community and for the general public. A regional Master Training program developed by Pinetree Institute is also in progress as part of this effort with over thirty Master Trainers deployed across the region to date.

Recommendations:
- Continued outreach to build capacity for resilience and positive childhood experiences.
- Continued development and delivery of education for target organizations.

2. Recovery Housing

Sober housing and transitional housing options are major gaps in the Portsmouth area, with currently no sober housing options available within Rockingham County. The full range of housing needs for individuals in recovery and transition needs considerable attention and no easy solutions are currently identified. This task force will further clarify current gaps and identify priorities for development for near- and long-term solutions.

Members:
Hon. Tina Nadeau, chair
Mark Lefebvre, Pinetree Institute, co-chair
Kim Bock, New Hampshire Coalition of Recovery Residences

Rachel Azotea, New Hampshire Judicial Branch
Kerry Norton, Hope on Haven Hill, advisor
Moné Cassier, Sober Sisters Recovery, advisor

Objectives:

- Evaluate state of Recovery Housing in the Seacoast.

- Research financial resources within New Hampshire.

- Evaluate best practices in other parts of the state.

- Establish relationship with New Hampshire Coalition of Recovery Residences.

- Issue report with findings and recommendations.

Needs: Sober housing and transitional housing options within Rockingham are needed to serve the greater Portsmouth area. Evidence has proven that stable and safe housing is one of the key factors in recovery. The full range of housing needs for individuals in recovery and transition needs considerable attention and no easy solutions are currently identified. This task force will further clarify current gaps and identify priorities for development for near- and long-term solutions.

Results: The Recovery Housing Task Force has reviewed the critical need for recovery housing in the area. At present, there is no recovery housing in all of Rockingham County. As a result, any individual in need of this support is referred out of the area, resulting in considerable barriers to achieving a positive recovery outcome. This task force has identified a range of grant and loan opportunities to support the development of recovery housing capacity and is currently working on a detailed plan to identify potential operators, sites, and the process forward to make this housing possible.

Over the last several months of 2020, seventy-nine applications for recovery housing from individuals within Rockingham County needed to be referred out of the county since there are currently no certified recovery residences in Rockingham County. There are many barriers to opening a recovery residence in the Seacoast, including the startup costs for potential operators and the stigma associated with individuals in recovery and residences that house these people. We find that although communities are generally supportive of recovery residences, members of these communities do not want them in their neighborhoods. Further barriers include a shortage of operators, prohibitive property values in the Seacoast, and a lack of available properties.

The task force did find that there are state and federal financial resources available in the form of grants, loans, and tax credits. As a way to mitigate some of these barriers, our advisors strongly suggest operating a recovery residence as a nonprofit entity and proactively working with communities and neighborhoods.

Grants—New Hampshire Community Development Finance Authority (CDFA)
- Grant money is available from the Community Development Block Grant (US HUD), which is administered by CDFA.
- CDFA also offers "planning grants" up to twenty-five thousand dollars.
- Grant money is also available from the Support Act.
- Tax Credits are available for donors as an incentive.

Loans—NH Housing Finance Authority
- Zero-interest, deferred loans as part of the Supportive Housing Program.
- Affordable Housing Fund (AHF)—appropriated by the state.
- Housing Trust Fund (HTF)—federally funded; state administered.

Recommendations:
- Establish a search committee to 1) seek a partnership of potential operators and 2) identify potential properties as a location.
- Conduct outreach to gain organizational support from local communities.
- Establish a planning group to investigate and apply for planning grant(s) and/or loans(s).

3. Employment

Finding employment after treatment and transition back into the workforce is a major issue for people attempting to manage a successful recovery. There are significant programs through organizations such as New Hampshire Works for Recovery, SOS Recovery Community Organization, Safe Harbor Recovery, and the Governor's Recovery Friendly Workplace program that are just now getting full attention in the Portsmouth area. This task force will work to ensure that these programs and others like it are being fully utilized and identify other areas in which support for employment can be augmented.

Members:
Mark Lefebvre, Pinetree Institute, co-chair
Elizabeth Miller, program manager, NH Works for Recovery
Mary Boisse, SOS Recovery Community Organization, co-chair

Jeanne Venuti, Governor's Recovery Friendly Workplace
Whitney Brown, Granite Pathways Job Launch Program
Valerie Rochon, president, Portsmouth Collaborative Chamber
Dana Lariviere, CEO, Chameleon Group

Objectives:
- Research and document the state of workforce development and training options available to individuals in recovery.

- Research and document the staffing trends and needs of local businesses given the impact of COVID.

- Develop an outreach program for employers seeking workers.

- Develop an outreach program for agencies and service providers regarding the available workforce development and educations services.

Needs: Prior to COVID, the committee focused on the needs of job seekers and employers in a labor market with a 6 percent unemployment rate in New Hampshire. As a result, our initial focus was to channel potential job seekers who are in recovery to the appropriate agencies in the region for job placement and training services. Further, we continued to reach out to employers who expressed interest in becoming a Recovery Friendly Workplace, a program that helps attract and retain workers who may be struggling with addiction.

The impact of COVID to the labor market and economy was devastating to New Hampshire businesses. As COVID restrictions became relaxed, businesses were now struggling to find workers. The focus has since returned to conducting outreach to job seekers and employers to inform them of the various education and employment services in the Seacoast region.

Results: Local workforce development services are available from Safe Harbor/Granite Pathways with the Job Launch program, Southern New Hampshire Services for the New Hampshire Works program, SOS Recovery Community Organization with peer recovery services and workforce development services, and the Governor's Recovery Friendly Workplace program. These programs continue to provide training, job placement, and peer recovery services to job seekers in the Portsmouth region. Further, these programs will offer qualified candidates education and technical assistance to employers seeking to recruit and retain employees in recovery.

Outreach and awareness campaigns continue with literature drops planned with the help of the Portsmouth Collaborative Chamber and promotional radio spots on WSCA Portsmouth Community Radio.

Recommendations:
- Continued outreach to employers to match job seekers with opportunities.
- Continued outreach to employers to promote the Governor's Recovery Friendly Workplace program and services.
- Continued outreach to job seekers to create awareness of and interest for education and employment services.
- Continued outreach to job seekers and employers to create awareness of peer recovery services.

Tip: When well-intentioned organizations and programs appear to overlap, invest in the time to clarify, and position these organizations within the coalition and to the public.

4. Access & Connectivity

Transportation was initially identified as a major gap with very few existing options. The underlying issue, we learned, is one of access in general. The transportation task force was originally charged with examining current options and exploring new options for transportation, especially in situations where individuals may not have a license or reliable access to a car. As a result of COVID, this task force shifted its focus to accessibility in general, and especially access to technology that would allow individuals to connect to online telehealth and tele-recovery services.

Members:
Cliff Lazenby, co-chair
Larry McCullough, Pinetree Institute, co-chair
Mark Lefebvre, Pinetree Institute
Alan Gold, Portsmouth Economic Development Commission

Objectives:
- Evaluate existing options for access to health, recovery, and other clinical and non-clinical services in the Seacoast.
- Evolve from a limited scope of transportation to identify gaps to providing voice, video, and digital connection via smartphones.
- Adapt to COVID-related restrictions on physical access to services.
- Conduct outreach and recruit partners to participate in a coordinated technology pilot.

Needs: Many people seeking recovery services lack smartphones and data plans to access clinical and non-clinical services. An existing phone distribution program in Strafford County Public Health Network provides a successful model to replicate in the greater Portsmouth area. The task force determined that a regional approach would be more effective than deployment within a single municipality.

Results: The team worked with T-Mobile and the Seacoast Public Health Network to provide mobile phones, a data plan, and access for an initial twelve- to eighteen-month period to those in recovery, all free of charge. The program, called "Seacoast Health Connect," launched in April and helps to close the gap for individuals needing access to telehealth, tele-recovery support, meetings, and other basic needs such as finding a job, housing, and reconnecting with family. We emphasized simple paperwork for agencies and phone recipients to participate.

Recommendations:
- Monitor usage to determine program effectiveness.
- Revisit progress in the future, continue funding if successful.

5. Coordination

Helping individuals in recovery navigate the complex maze of services and eligibility requirements is a significant need for individuals and families impacted by addiction. The Doorway in Dover, New Hampshire, is one attempt to address this issue, but we learned that the Portsmouth area is still greatly underserved by the Dover Doorway. This task force addressed the issue of care coordination that includes approaches to case management and also explored issues related to shared information, service planning, and access to services.

Members:
Justin Looser, Portsmouth Regional Hospital, co-chair
Mark Lefebvre, Pinetree Institute, co-chair
Peter Fifield, The Doorway
Dustin Ward, Safe Harbor Recovery Center
Rebecca Throop, Seacoast Mental Health Center

Objectives:
- Evaluate existing coordination approaches for both clinical and non-clinical services in the Seacoast.

- Research existing tools for coordination in New Hampshire.

- Evaluate best practices in other parts of the state.

- Recommend a coordination platform for Portsmouth area.

- Conduct outreach and recruit partners to participate in selected coordination platform.

Needs: Individuals seeking addiction services often find it difficult to navigate the network of providers in a timely fashion. Once they are in the ecosystem of providers, the system often lacks a coordinated system of hand-off from one provider to another. This results in missed appointments, lack of visibility of outcomes, and gaps in service coverage.

Results: The Doorway is the hub for coordination of services in the Seacoast and has recently expanded into the Seacoast region at the SOS Hampton location at 1 Lafayette Road. Unite Us (www.uniteus.com) has been selected by the New Hampshire Department of Health and Human Services (DHHS) as a coordination software platform, and the Doorway has adopted this platform for regional coordination.

Since the Unite Us implementation dovetails nicely with the needs and timing of the Coordination task force, we have adopted a networking model based on this platform initiative. The software connects those in need of help with navigating access to resources such as the Department of Employment Security, the Department of Health and Human Services, Medicaid, and networks of peer support services.

Recommendations:
- It is recommended that coalition continue on the path to adopt the Unite Us platform under the leadership of the Doorway.

- It is recommended that the task force focus its energy on building a robust network of registered Unite Us partners through outreach and education.

Phase 2 Summary

In closing, the Portsmouth Coordinated Response to Substance Use Disorder delivered tangible results to the community. Five task forces were established, and each conducted in-depth research on current capacity across priority focus areas: Community Education, Housing, Employment, Access, and Coordination. Recommendations were made to the steering committee on ways to increase capacity where required. In addition to these efforts continuing forward, the steering committee is recommending an expansion to the regional focus with the launch of the Seacoast Coordinated Response to SUD with local focus not only on Portsmouth, but neighboring communities of Hampton, Exeter, and Seabrook. A proposal outlining this Seacoast Coordinated Response has been developed and is being shared with relevant regional and local stakeholders.

> **Tip:** Assign at least one non-facilitator as co-chair; rotate co-chair assignment to other task force members. This would ensure that the content emerging from each of the task forces is not interpreted as the point of view of the facilitating organization.

Phase 3: Design & Implementation (2021-2022)

At the end of Phase 2 of the Portsmouth Coordinated Response to SUD, the committee recommended an expansion to a regional focus with the launch of the Seacoast Coordinated Response to SUD with local focus on the communities of Portsmouth, Hampton, Exeter, and Seabrook. This section summarizes the findings and recommendations following the expansion to the Seacoast Coordinated Response, and of each task force as described below.

In October 2021, we convened an in-person gathering of Hampton leaders across key community sectors to share the findings of the Portsmouth Coordinated Response and introduce the concept of a community-coordinated approach to these sector leaders. The outcome of that meeting was the commitment of these sector leaders to participate on the Seacoast Coordinated Response, representing the town of Hampton.

The members of the *Portsmouth Steering Committee* as of October 2021 were as follows. It is notable that as elected officials change or former members have moved on to other opportunities, that the coalition has adapted accordingly.

- **City Government:** Deaglan McEachern, mayor
- **City Manager:** Karen Conard
- **Department of Public Health:** Kim McNamara, health officer
- **New Hampshire State Senate:** Rebecca Perkins Kwoka, District 21
- **The Doorway:** Pete Fifield
- **Courts:** Hon. Tina Nadeau, chief justice
- **Child Advocacy:** Maureen Sullivan, executive director, Child Advocacy Center of Rockingham County
- **Greater Seacoast Community Health:** Lara Drolet, chief strategy officer
- **Corrections:** Jessica Norton, Rockingham County Director of Inmate Services/ Programming

- **Law Enforcement:** Cpt. Darrin Sargent; Lt. David Keaveny; Chief Mark Newport (ex officio)

- **Fire/First Responders:** Chief William McQuillen

- **School Unit:** Christine Burke, wellness director; Stephen Zadravec, superintendent (ex officio)

- **Hospital:** Justin Looser, administrative market director

- **Recovery Centers:** Whitney Brown, Safe Harbor Recovery Center Director; Erica Ungarelli, Granite Pathways director

- **Domestic/Sexual Abuse:** Sarah Shanahan, program director

- **Housing:** Tammy Joslyn, residential services coordinator, Portsmouth Housing Authority

- **Chamber of Commerce:** Ben VanCamp, Chamber Collaborative of Greater Portsmouth

- **Seacoast Public Health Network:** Maria Reyes, Continuum of Care coordinator

- **Economic Development:** Alan Gold, Portsmouth, vice chair, Portsmouth EDC

- **Mental Health Services:** Seacoast Mental Health Center: Diane Fontneau, clinical manager, SUD Program; Patty Driscoll, vice president of clinical operations, Adult Services

- **Facilitation & Coordination:** Pinetree Institute: Dr. Larry McCullough, executive director; Mark Lefebvre, director of community engagement; Elizabeth Miller, program director

The members of the *Hampton Steering Committee* as of July 2021 are listed below:

- **Hampton Town Selectmen:** Rusty Bridle, Jim Waddell

- **New Hampshire State Senate:** Dr. Tom Sherman, New Hampshire State Senator, District 24

- **Hampton Police Department:** David Hobbs, chief; Richard Sawyer, former chief

- **Hampton Fire Department:** Michael McMahon, chief

- **Hampton School Department:** Dean Millard, School of Trades

- **Hampton Area Chamber of Commerce:** John Nyhan, president

- **SOS Recovery:** John Burns, director

- **Recovery Housing:** Jules Johnson, director of Magnolia House

Seabrook and Exeter Coalitions

Despite multiple attempts to convene community leaders and decision makers in both Seabrook and Exeter, we were not able to gain enough traction to expand the coalition into these two communities. However, since many of the providers and services of the Seacoast area are regional, both Seabrook and Exeter benefited from the work of the coalition.

1. Community Education and Training Task Force

The committee agreed there is a need for more preventive educational programs for families, children, and youth including social-emotional learning and specific substance use disorder understanding that this task force will address. One of the top needs identified is for greater awareness and training on the topic of adverse childhood experiences (ACEs) and trauma-informed care both for the professional service community and for the general public. Several initiatives are underway including a Master Training program being implemented by Pinetree Institute.

Results:
- Over three hundred individuals have received free ACEs training.
- Developed a Prevention Services Database of youth-serving organizations in the community.
- This task force has transitioned to the Greater Portsmouth Youth Wellness Coalition in order to mobilize the community to prevent and reduce substance use among youth by creating sustainable, community-level change.

Recommendations:
- Continue outreach to build capacity for resilience and positive childhood experiences.
- Continue with the development and delivery of education for target organizations.
- Continue transition to the Greater Portsmouth Youth Wellness Coalition.

2. Recovery Housing Task Force

Sober housing and transitional housing options continue to be major gaps in the Seacoast region of New Hampshire. Until October 2021 there were no sober housing options available within Rockingham County.

Results: The Recovery Housing Task Force reviewed the critical need for recovery housing in the area. At the outset of our efforts, there was no recovery housing in all of Rockingham County. Until recently, all individuals in need of this support are referred out of the area, resulting in considerable challenges to a positive recovery outcome.

Although outside of the operation of the Seacoast Coordinated Response to SUD initiative, Magnolia House opened in Hampton, New Hampshire, with twelve beds for women. The operator of Magnolia House, Jules Johnson, opened Summerwood House in Hampton with twelve beds for men. Summerwood House was opened under the leadership of the Seacoast Coordinated Response initiative whereby an anonymous donor, a local property developer, and Jules Johnson as the operator made this possible. Where we had zero beds in Rockingham County at the start of this phase of the Greater Portsmouth Recovery Coalition, we closed out with twelve beds for men and another twelve beds for women.

Recommendations:
- Evaluate the need for alternative/progressive "levels" of housing in the region (as described by New Hampshire Coalition of Recovery Residence).

- Evaluate the need of recovery housing for underserved populations such as veterans, LGBTQ+, justice-involved, women with children, men with children, BIPOC, etc.

3. Employment Task Force

Employment after treatment and transition back into the workforce continues to be a major issue for people attempting to manage a successful recovery. Employers are also seeking training and services for employees within their organizations either directly or indirectly affected by SUD. There are significant programs through organizations such as SOS Recovery Community Organization, Safe Harbor Recovery, and the Governor's Recovery Friendly Workplace program that continue to operate in the Seacoast area.

Results: Workforce development services are available from Safe Harbor/Granite Pathways with the Job Launch program; Southern New Hampshire Services for the New Hampshire Works program, SOS Recovery Community Organization with peer recovery services and workforce development services, and the Governor's Recovery Friendly Workplace program. These programs will continue to provide training, job placement, and recovery services to job seekers in the Portsmouth region. Further, these programs will offer qualified candidates, education, and technical assistance to employers seeking to recruit and retain employees in recovery.

New Hampshire Community Colleges offer WorkReadyNH programming for "soft skill" development. Great Bay Community College now participates on this task force.

Outreach and awareness campaigns continue with literature drops planned with the help of the Portsmouth Collaborative Chamber and promotional radio spots on WSCA Portsmouth Community Radio.

Recommendations:
- Continued outreach to employers to match job seekers with opportunities.
- Continued outreach to employers to promote the Governor's Recovery Friendly Workplace program and services.
- Continued outreach to job seekers to create awareness of and interest for education and employment services.
- Continued outreach to job seekers and employers to create awareness of peer recovery services.
- Continued collaboration with Business and Industry Association of New Hampshire, local Chambers of Commerce, and local businesses to address barriers for prospective and current workers.
- Expand collaboration with Great Bay Community College for WorkReadyNH programs.

4. Access & Connectivity Task Force

For several months, this task force continued to support the Seacoast Health Connect program of distributing smartphones to individuals lacking the means to access their providers, families, and other services. This task force shifted its focus to accessibility and technology that would allow individuals to connect to online telehealth and tele-recovery services. It should be noted that this program was terminated in early 2022 due to lack of capacity to administer this program.

Recommendations:
- Survey the community to determine if the telehealth program would still be effective, and if so, seek a program administrator.
- Revisit transportation as an issue with the steering committee.

> **TIP:** When a program or service is not meeting its objectives, or if situations arise where delivery of that program or service can no longer be supported, don't be afraid to adapt and move on to serve another need.

5. Coordination of Services Task Force:

Results: Unite Us tracked statewide results and the Seacoast region proved to be an effective use of their platform. Results as of July 2022:

- New Hampshire organization with the most inbound referrals: The Doorway of Dover
- Top network need: substance use disorder services
- Total in-network organizations serving residents in the Seacoast: fifty-six
- Top organizations by Service Type: substance use disorder

Recommendations:

- It is recommended the coalition continue on the path to grow the United Us platform under the leadership of the Doorway through outreach.

Phase 3: Summary

The Portsmouth Coordinated Response to Substance Use Disorder delivered tangible results to the community. During this phase, the coalition attempted an expansion with a regional focus with the launch of the Seacoast Coordinated Response to SUD. This effort required local commitments from the individual communities of Portsmouth, Hampton, Exeter, and Seabrook. Although Seabrook and Exeter were not in a state of readiness for such a coalition, Hampton did indeed embrace the model and, as a result, opened the very first men's recovery home in Rockingham County.

In July 2023, the Portsmouth Coordinated Response to SUD convened to discuss the Phase 3 results. While we were successful in our efforts to integrate the town of Hampton into the Seacoast Coordinated Response coalition, we were not as successful expanding to the towns of Seabrook and Exeter. After multiple unsuccessful efforts to convene a group of sector leaders, we realized that Exeter and Seabrook did not yet have the capacity to take on a coalition. Therefore, this phase of Seacoast Coordinated Response to SUD focused primarily on Portsmouth and Hampton area communities.

That said, and despite the lack of sector participation for Exeter and Seabrook to join the Seacoast Coordinated Response initiative, residents of both communities continue to benefit from the work of the task forces, which by nature are regionally focused.

> **Tip:** Do not pursue community-wide coalitions where communities do not have enough initial capacity or the necessary commitment to come to the table. Focus on those sectors individually that are prepared to build that initial capacity. Come back to the community level at a later time.

Recommendation to the Steering Committee

1. Schedule a working session with extended team (including task forces) to confirm existing priorities and consider others that have emerged since the coalition's inception.

2. Extend the scope of this coalition to establish Portsmouth as a Recovery Ready Community.

Decision: Expansion and Rebranding—The Greater Portsmouth Recovery Coalition

The Portsmouth Coordinated Response Steering Committee met in July 2022, to review the results of the design and implementation phases of the Portsmouth Coordinated Response to SUD. In addition to the steering committee, several members of the five task forces were also present.

After reviewing the results of Phase 3 and a spirited discussion on next steps, there was overwhelming support for the recommendations of the task forces. The leadership team posed three questions to the group before breaking up into workgroups:

1. What do we continue doing?

2. What do we stop doing?

3. What do we do differently?

The consensus answer to the question of what areas the coalition should consider discontinuing was none. Further, in response to the question about what we should do differently, the coalition identified other areas to consider:

1. Increase community awareness and education to reduce stigma.

2. Define and measure outcomes.

3. Address mental health and substance use disorders as co-occurring illnesses.

4. Assess harm reduction needs and capabilities.

5. Extend services to homeless populations.

6. Include youth as a population.

7. Move upstream to prevention.

Most notable was the extension of the coalition's mission to achieve the goal of establishing Portsmouth as a *Recovery Ready Community*. The results of the prior three years of coalition have proven that a coordinated response model—having sector representation, gaining community commitment to the cause, and investing in neutral facilitation—works. The coalition was well-positioned to respond to the expanding needs of the Portsmouth community to achieve its vision of becoming a Recovery Ready Community.

Phase 4: Continued Implementation and Evaluation (2022–2024)

By January 2023, the coalition had completed a preliminary inventory of needs, existing services and priorities for the new task forces added to the coalition's mission. The exceptions were Programming for Youth and Prevention workgroups that were integrated into the Greater Portsmouth Youth Wellness Coalition. That coalition eventually applied for and was awarded a CDC Drug-Free Community Grant.

Services for Homeless
- **Exists:** Cross Roads House, community warming centers, Hope on Haven Hill, New Generation, Families First, Seacoast Mental Health, Seacoast Pathways, Safe Harbor Recovery Center.
- **Needs:** Veterans' services, more outreach workers, mobile health van, media coverage, bringing resources and services to people, check-ins, housing (recovery, public, temporary), wrap-around services.
- **Priorities:** Quantify scope of the issue, coordination and joining of participating providers, funding.

Marketing/Media Relations
- **Exists:** Great local marketing and PR agencies and talent (Brown & Company Design, DARCI Creative, Boldwerks, Rumbletree), partnerships at Drug Free NH, community and public radio/TV, marketing directors at social service agencies, public affairs office of the city.
- **Needs:** Name and logo, social media plan, PR outreach calendar, success stories, impact reports.
- **Priorities:** Recruitment for this team

Co-Occurring Disorders

- **Exists:** Seacoast Mental Health, Families First, Seacoast Youth Services, Addiction Recovery Services, Portsmouth Behavioral Health.

- **Needs:** Co-occurring partial hospitalization (PHP), low-barrier psychiatric/MAT/MOUD, case managers/community navigators, reimbursement rates vs. cost of services, re-entry services for justice-involved, training

- **Priorities:** Recruitment for this team

Harm Reduction

- **Exists:** Syringe Services Programs (SSP), disposal services, educational materials, distribution methods.

- **Need:** Community education (stigma, mindset change), resource guide/navigator—"know who, what, where, how, when"

- **Priorities:** Recruitment for this team, strategy/plan

In July 2023, the coalition steering committee and task force members met to review the first six months of this phase of the coalition. What was made clear at this quarterly coalition meeting was that the coalition membership was expanding, and that providers were stepping up their efforts to bring much needed services to the greater Portsmouth area. At that time nearly seventy individuals from nearly forty-five organizations were participating in the Greater Portsmouth Recovery Coalition.

The notable accomplishments thus far included:

- Harm Reduction services were provided at Safe Harbor Recovery Center under the leadership of New Hampshire Harm Reduction Coalition.

- Education & Awareness campaigns for Harm Reduction, Recovery Housing, and Workforce Development underway.

- Services for homeless individuals and families at Safe Harbor Recovery Center and Cross Roads House under the leadership of Families First.

- Research underway for a sustainable funding model for Recovery Housing in the Seacoast.

- Created a Marketing & Community Education blog and social media presence for the coalition.

- Workforce Development task force members Safe Harbor Job Launch, New Hampshire Recovery Friendly Workplace, Working Fields and WorkReadyNH appearance at 3S Artspace Collaborative Chamber of Greater Portsmouth event.

- Workforce Development is conducting a survey of Chamber Collaborative of Greater Portsmouth members regarding their knowledge of the area workforce development programs.

- The Marketing & Community Education task force is hosting a film screening of *Our American Family* on September 21 at 3S Artspace.

- Families First providing primary and mental health services at Cross Roads House and soon at Safe Harbor Recovery Center under the Access to Services task force.

- Better Life Partners and Groups Recovery Together offering Medication-Assisted Treatment (MAT) under the Access to Services task force.

- The Co-Occurring Disorder task force identified the need for more training/awareness for SUD and Mental Health providers—New Hampshire Alcohol and Drug Abuse Counselors Association (NHADACA) to provide new training offerings.

- The Co-Occurring Disorder task force members will collaborate with New Hampshire Recovery Friendly Workplace to develop training content for businesses under the RFW program.

- The Systems, Data & Reporting task force has identified desired outcomes to measure progress across the coalition.

In September 2023, I was reassigned to direct the Maine statewide Recovery Friendly Workplace program, and Molly Louison-Semrow took over the role of leading the Greater Portsmouth Recovery Coalition. She continues in this role today with Meghan Stewart as program coordinator and Brandi Lee as program administrator.

At the end of 2023, I retired from Pinetree Institute to focus on producing the podcast series, *It Takes A Village: Addiction Prevention & Recovery on the Seacoast,*[245] and the writing of this book. One of the first interviews I conducted for the podcast series was with Molly, which focused on her thoughts from her first six months working with the coalition.

"One of the big areas we put our effort in during recent months is to develop strong and unified mission statements, objectives, purposes, and to introduce a new tool to track coalition outcomes," she said. "What I saw was a group of incredibly passionate people that wanted to help however they could, and they were in the right task forces. But the beauty of being a coalition leader is that it's not about us, it's not about the facilitating agency. If we're doing our jobs, we should be uplifting everyone else."[246]

I asked her, "Is there some aspect or accomplishment of the Greater Portsmouth Recovery Coalition that stands out from the rest?"

"Yes. I can't say enough about Portsmouth public health department's commitment to harm reduction, they have been a fantastic partner," Molly said. "They willingly got much of their staff trained with the New Hampshire Harm Reduction Coalition and Safe Harbor. And most recently, they had a great idea, which was to open up their offices as a naloxone distribution site during that same time, since some people may prefer a private office setting or that were not comfortable, for whatever reason, going to a recovery center. This has been a great idea, because we want as many outlets as possible for people to get safe use supplies, and for people to get overdose prevention supplies. They are really champions of this work, the city of Portsmouth, and that has been led by their own initiative. They certainly have not been dragged along the way with this project. This happened under the leadership of Director Kim McNamara and her staff at the city of Portsmouth Department of Public Health."

Phase 5: Sustained Collaboration (2024–)

Larry McCullough bristled at the term I proposed for the current state of the Greater Portsmouth Recovery Coalition. I suggested that in its fifth year, the coalition is in "maintenance" mode. "Nope," he said, "too passive."

I can't recall if it was Larry or I who suggested the term *Sustained Collaboration*, but that term seemed to resonate. I think I came up with the word sustained, and he suggested collaboration. Molly concurred.

The struggle we were having centered around Pinetree Institute's changing role as facilitator of the coalition. The membership and the task forces are still going strong with measured progress against a predetermined set of outcomes that were democratically proposed by the task force members themselves. There's something organic about self-determination in this context of community building and community-driven solutions to a public health crisis.

Pinetree Institute's role as the facilitator of the coalition is evolving, but the coalition abides. To that end, Pinetree continues to host and regularly document meetings for the coalition membership for information sharing. Progress against outcomes are discussed. Where help is needed at the task force level, help is provided as the network connection among coalition partners remains strong.

The Greater Portsmouth Recovery Coalition will continue to build recovery capacity in the community. Plans include establishing a community of practice (CoP), with meeting minutes, a forum for online discussion, and sharing of best practices. And based on the strength of the coalition, we have built a rapid-response capability should a crisis emerge.

As a direct result of the Greater Portsmouth Recovery Coalition's efforts, the community now has harm reduction, medication-assisted treatment, recovery housing, multiple workforce development programs, community awareness of ACEs and PCEs, trauma-informed care, a podcast series, services for unhoused populations, training for co-occurring disorders, and re-entry services for the justice involved.

EPILOGUE

I often think back to that day in August 2012, when I was about to be discharged from Portsmouth Regional Hospital's Behavioral Health Unit—clueless, hopeless, and unsure about my future. Whisked off to Logan Airport by my wife with a one-way ticket ("Don't come back until you're ready to come back") and a hastily packed suitcase in the back seat, we made that ride in awkward silence. Neither one of us had any clue as to what the future held for each of us as individuals and as a couple.

In hindsight, I know now that I was one of the fortunate ones. I had the financial means to go to treatment, albeit out of state, to a program that was recommended based on the experience of a family friend. I was able to get the professional treatment that likely saved my life.

Portsmouth Regional Hospital did not have an aftercare case worker to make calls on my behalf. They did not have a resource center for me to research programs in the area because there were no programs in the area. My discharge documents included a book of Alcoholics Anonymous meetings and my medical diagnosis of generalized anxiety disorder, major depressive disorder, and polysubstance disorder. I was to follow up with my general physician.

If I were to be discharged today from the same unit, I would have an aftercare program that included a referral to one of the several treatment centers within the state. It would have a contact for me to call at Safe Harbor Recovery Center to assist me with my recovery journey. I'd have a referral to a prescribing doctor or nurse practitioner for medicated assisted treatment. If I needed a ride, one would be provided by a volunteer from Safe Harbor Recovery Center. If I needed harm reduction services, I had multiple options locally as a result of the New Hampshire Harm Reduction Coalition. If I needed a peer recovery coach, I had several options to meet with one. If I needed an intensive outpatient program following residential treatment, I could find one at either Addiction Recovery Services or Seacoast Mental Health. If I was homeless, there was a Families First van to provide me with medical services. Safe Harbor would provide me with supplies if I lived in a tent encampment. If I needed a case worker to get me entered into the appropriate level of care today, I could call 2-1-1 and enter the Doorway. If my family needed assistance today, NAMI New Hampshire, Seacoast Mental Health, Families First, and Safe Harbor all offer programs and support.

The Seacoast area of New Hampshire was a desert when it came to recovery-sustaining services in 2012. There is still a lot of work to do, like implementing community recovery navigators and increasing the capacity of recovery housing. However, thanks to the Greater Portsmouth Recovery Coalition, and the seeds planted by a small but representative group of community leaders, the community has shown the will and the commitment to make these things happen. Portsmouth today is a shining example of a Recovery Ready Community.

APPENDIX

Templates

Building Coalitions

Coalition Checklist			
Organizational Checklist	**Name**	**Organization**	**Decision Maker? Y/N**
People with Lived Experience			
People in Recovery			
People Who Use Drugs			
Family Members			
Treatment			
Inpatient Treatment			
Outpatient Treatment			
Co-occurring SUD and Mental Health Providers			
MAT Providers			
Harm Reduction Providers			
Recovery			
Recovery Community Organization			
Peer Recovery Coach			
Recovery Housing			
Recovery Workforce			
Re-Entry			
Municipality			
City/Town Government			
First Responders			
Law Enforcement			
Schools			
Other			
Hospital			
Chamber of Commerce			
Judicial			
Local Media			
DEI Representation			
Community Action Programs			
Mutual Aid (AA, NA, Al-Anon)			
Faith Community			
Facilitating Organization			

Memorandum of Understanding (MOU)

Memorandum of Understanding

Between [COALITION] and [MEMBER]: _____

Mission

The mission of [COALITION] is to [. . .]

EXAMPLE: The mission of this coalition is to create sustainable well-being for individuals, families, and our communities. Together, the parties enter this Memorandum of Understanding to mutually promote healthy communities by providing addiction recovery support and services for individuals and families in our community.

Purpose and Scope

[COALITION] and [MEMBER] both work to [. . .]

EXAMPLE: The purpose of this coalition is to promote recovery and serve individuals and families in recovery and/or facing barriers to accessing recovery services. Our organizations are committed to improving the health of communities and individuals throughout our community. Working collaboratively, we can advance our mission effectively and efficiently. This MOU outlines the expectations of both parties as it relates to this program funding:

    A. [COALITION] will provide:

        a. _____

        b. _____

    B. [MEMBER] will provide:

        a. _____

        b. _____

Terms of Understanding

This MOU is effective upon [DATE or EVENT] for the duration of [TIME PERIOD]. Insert other provisions as appropriate.

Authorization

I agree to the terms outlined herein:

_____   _____
NAME   NAME

_____   _____
ROLE, TITLE   ROLE, TITLE

Logic Model

Resources/ Inputs	Activities	Output	Short Term Outcomes	Intermediate Outcomes	Long-Term Outcomes

Recovery Ready Checklist

Minimal Elements of a Recovery Ready Community	
1. Youth Programing	
2. Harm Reduction	
3. Community Education & Outreach	
4. Medication-Assisted Treatment	
5. In-Patient Treatment	
6. Out-Patient Treatment	
7. Treatment Courts	
8. Recovery Housing	
9. Recovery Community Organizations	
10. Recovery Employment	
11. Access to Services	
12. Re-Entry Services	
13. Peer Recovery Coaches	
14. Recovery Community Navigator	

RESOURCES

Tamarack Institute Coalition Sustainability Toolkit

https://www.tamarackcommunity.ca/sustainability-and-resilience
-resource-library

Commonly Well: Recovery Capital Index

https://commonlywell.com/the-recovery-capital-index-a-validated
-assessment/

Recovery Ready Community Outcomes (Kentucky)

https://rrcky.org/

National Recovery-Ready Workplace Toolkit

https://www.dol.gov/agencies/eta/RRW-hub/Toolkit

**Getting Started–Pinetree Institute Recovery Ready
Community Practice**

https://pinetreeinstitute.org

ACKNOWLEDGMENTS

A special note of gratitude to the insanely talented Eric Ott, who was generous with his time and talents and patient with the author. I will be forever grateful for his gifts.

Deidre Randall and Peter E. Randall Publisher for believing in me.

Mayor Deaglan McEachern and Cliff Lazenby for their leadership.

Family and Friends

Vivian, Joey, and Selena Lefebvre
Steven and Andrea Martin
Stephen and Laurie Belmonte
Danielle DeYeso
Michael DeYeso
Colleen Giambarresi
Mark and Julie Bucceri
Michelle Buccheri
Tony and Donna Lefebvre
Mike and Kim Lefebvre
Patricia Aubuchon Lefebvre

Pinetree Institute

Larry McCullough, Molly Louison-Semrow, Brandi Lee, Brittany Reichmann, Meaghan Stewart, Amy Michaels, Autumn Allen, Catherine Rawson, Alan Gold, Gregg Dowty, Danielle Nonamacher, Ann Bliss, Kim Kelsey

Greater Portsmouth Recovery Coalition

Martha Fuller Clark, Hon. Tina Nadeau, Maureen Sullivan, Stephen Church, Robert Merner, Darrin Sargent, Todd Germain, Stephen Zadravec, Christine Burke, Alan Gold, Grant Turpin, Stephen Curtis, Jay Couture, Diane Fontneau, Heather Blumenfeld, Patricia Reed, Kathy Beebe, Sarah Shanahan, Tammy Joslyn, Valerie Rachon, State Senator Rebecca Perkins Kwoka, Jessica Norton, Justin Looser, Dustin Ward, Rebecca Throop, Rachel Azotea, Kerry Norton, Mone Cassier, Elizabeth Miller, Jeanne Venuti, Whitney Brown, Dana Lariviere, Karen Morton Clark, Peter Fifield, Nadine Lamontagne,

Kim Bock, Jules Johnson, Mary Boisse, Ben VanCamp, Patrice Baker, Lara Drolet, Karen Conard, Maria Reyes, Kim McNamara, Lauren McGinley, Neal Ouellett, Zach McLaughlin, William McQuillen, Erica Ungarelli, Patty Driscoll, Sandra Beaudry, Will Arvelo, Mary Beth Hardy, Patte Ardizonni, Dawn Hamdi, Emily Carrara, Stephanie Jordan, Crystal Pomeroy, Sarah Fetras, Justin Younger, Lynn Kearney, Jillian Kurtz, Freddy Petrone, Nicole Seaward, Kati Pittendreigh, Darci Knowles, Julie Yerkes, Monte Bohanan, Coreen Toussaint, Ellen Tully, Missy Leeman, John Iudice, Karen Frarie, Emily Kannenberg, Christine Burke, Deb Grabowski, Joanna Diemer, Ellen Tully, Liz Baude, Suzanne Weete

Strafford County Addiction Task Force

Ashley Wheeler, Cora Long

Lewiston-Auburn

Jennifer Edwards, Rowan McFadden, Catherine Ryder, Betty Bartos

York County/Kennebunk Coordinated Response to SUD

Robert McKenzie, Liz Torrance, Jamie Baburek, Cheri Sullivan, Brad Paige, Mike Pardue, Bill King, Dr. Jessika Morin, Alyssa Pelchat, Jenna Ingram, Tricia Cote, Lacey Bailey, Carolyn Delaney, Diane Small

Town of Hampton

Rusty Bridle, Dr. and State Senator Tom Sherman, David Hobbs, Richard Sawyer, Michael McMahon, Dave O'Connor, Dean Millard, John Nyhan, Jim Waddell, Josh Yazgan, Stephanie Bergeron-Yazgan, Al Fleury

Town of Exeter

Jennifer Wheeler, Jennifer McGowan, Kathy Flygare

Seacoast Youth Service

Vic Maloney, Stephanie Wright, Sarah Fetras, Janine Richards

WSCA Portsmouth Community Radio

Nicole Seaward, Robbie McCluskey, Cantey Smith, Miles Bebbington, Rebecca Ingalls

Chase Home

Meme Wheeler, Lily Cragg, Ashley Murphy

Advisors

Seth Kaplan, Sam Quinones, David Best, David Whitesock, Aaron Williams, Eliza Zarka, Anena Hansen, Lisa Attygalle, Dr. Alex Elswick, Laura Pratt, Gordon Smith, Samantha Lewandowski, Denyse Richter, Lara Merchant, Danielle Parent, Alison Jones Webb, Robin Rieske, Chelsea Bardot Lewis, Leslie Clark, Eli George, Dr. Tom Sherman

NOTES

1   Substance Abuse and Mental Health Services Administration, *Results from the 2012 National Survey on Drug Use and Health: Summary of National Findings*, NSDUH Series H-46, HHS Publication No. (SMA) 13-4795. Rockville, MD: Substance Abuse and Mental Health Services Administration, 2013.

2   Substance Abuse and Mental Health Services Administration. (2023). *Key substance use and mental health indicators in the United States: Results from the 2022 National Survey on Drug Use and Health* (HHS Publication No. PEP23-07-01-006, NSDUH Series H-58). Center for Behavioral Health Statistics and Quality, Substance Abuse and Mental Health Services Administration. https://www.samhsa.gov/data/report/2022-nsduh-annual-national-report.

3   Weiland, Noah. "U.S. Recorded Nearly 110,000 Overdose Deaths in 2022," *New York Times*, May 17, 2023, https://www.nytimes.com/2023/05/17/us/politics/drug-overdose-deaths.html.

4   Ibid.

5   New Hampshire Drug Monitoring Initiative. "December 2023 Report," New Hampshire Information & Analysis Center, January 30, 2024, https://www.dhhs.nh.gov/sites/g/files/ehbemt476/files/documents2/dmi-dec2023.pdf.

6   Gokee, Amanda, Porter, Steven. "A Closer Look at the Recent Decline in Overdose Deaths in N.H.," *Boston Globe*, February 29, 2024, https://www.bostonglobe.com/2024/02/29/metro/closer-look-recent-decline-overdose-deaths-nh/.

7   Lawlor, Joe. "Drug Overdose Deaths Declined by 16% in Maine in 2023," *Portland Press Herald*, February 2, 2024, https://www.pressherald.com/2024/02/02/drug-overdose-deaths-down-16-in-maine-in-2023/.

8   Centers for Disease Control. "Stop Overdose: Fentanyl Facts," Accessed September, 28, 2024, https://www.cdc.gov/stopoverdose/index.html.

9   Quinones, Sam. "The fentanyl crisis is being driven by supply—not demand," *Washington Post*, January 31, 2024, https://www.washingtonpost.com/opinions/2024/01/31/fentanyl-opioid-epidemic-supply-demand/.

10   Quinones, Sam. "Only one thing will solve the fentanyl crisis," *Washington Post*, March 21, 2023 https://www.washingtonpost.com/opinions/2023/03/21/fentanyl-methamphetamine-us-mexico-diplomacy/.

11   Drug Enforcement Agency, "One Pill Can Kill," Accessed September 28, 2024, https://www.dea.gov/onepill.

12   Quinones, Sam. *The Least of Us: True Tales in America and Hope in the Time of Fentanyl and Meth* (Bloomsbury Publishing, 2021), 367.

13   U.S. Department of Health and Human Services (HHS), Office of the Surgeon General, *Facing Addiction in America: The Surgeon General's Report on Alcohol, Drugs, and Health*. Washington, DC: HHS, November 2016.

14   Ibid.

15   NIDA. 2023, May 30. Preface. Retrieved from https://nida.nih.gov/research-topics/addiction-science/drugs-brain-behavior-science-of-addiction on December 19, 2023.

16   American Society of Addiction Medicine, *The ASAM National Practice Guideline for the Treatment of Opioid Use Disorder*, 2020.

17   American Psychiatric Association, *Diagnostic and Statistical Manual of Mental Disorders (5th edition)*. Washington: American Psychiatric Association, 2013.

18   NIDA. 2023, May 30. Preface. Retrieved from https://nida.nih.gov/research-topics/addiction-science/drugs-brain-behavior-science-of-addiction on December 19, 2023.

19   Jamison, Leslie. *The Recovery: Intoxication and Its Aftermath.* Little Brown and Company, 2018, 112.

20   John Iudice, guest, *It Takes a Village: Addiction Prevention & Recovery on the Seacoast* podcast series, episode 3, February 15, 2024.

21   Ibid.

22   Fletcher, Ernie, "Living the Dream," *Recovery—The Official Newsletter of the Fletcher Group Rural Center of Excellence,* 50 (May 2024).

23   John Iudice, guest, *It Takes a Village: Addiction Prevention & Recovery on the Seacoast* podcast series, episode 3, February 15, 2024.

24   Kakko, J., H. Alho, A. Baldacchino, R. Molina, F. A. Nava, and G. Shaya, "Craving in Opioid Use Disorder: From Neurobiology to Clinical Practice," *Frontiers in Psychiatry 10* (August 30, 2019): 592, https://doi.org/10.3389/fpsyt.2019.00592.

25   Author interview with Brittany Reichmann, March 9, 2024.

26   Maté, Gabor, *In the Realm of Hungry Ghosts: Close Encounters with Addiction* (London: Vermilion, 2018), 38.

27   Bessel A. van der Kolk, *The Body Keeps the Score: Brain, Mind, and Body in the Healing of Trauma.* New York: Viking, 2014.

28   SAMHSA Strategic Prevention Technical Assistance Center. *Adverse Childhood Experiences and the Role of Substance Misuse Prevention.* n.d.

29   Tolle, Eckhart. *The Power of Now: A Guide to Spiritual Enlightenment.* Novato, CA: New World Library, 2004, 23.

30   Maté, Gabor, *In the Realm of Hungry Ghosts: Close Encounters with Addiction.* London, UK: Vermilion, 2018, 272.

31   American Psychiatric Association, *Diagnostic and Statistical Manual of Mental Disorders (5th edition)*. Washington: American Psychiatric Association, 2013.

32   Substance Abuse and Mental Health Services Administration. "2022 National Survey on Drug Use and Health (NSDUH) Releases." Accessed September 30, 2024. https://www.samhsa.gov/data/release/2022-national-survey-drug-use-and-health-nsduh-releases.

33   John Iudice, guest, *It Takes a Village: Addiction Prevention & Recovery on the Seacoast* podcast series, episode 3, February 15, 2024.

34   Diane Fontneau, guest, *It Takes a Village: Addiction Prevention & Recovery on the Seacoast* podcast series, episode 11, June 14, 2024.

35   "Anonymous Interview." *Thanks for Asking* podcast series, episode 2, November 2020.

36   WKYT News Staff. "Chilling 911 Call: Mom Finds Son Overdosed, Using Call to Raise Awareness." *WKYT*, September 22, 2016. Accessed September 30, 2024. https://www.wkyt.com/content/news/Chilling-911-call-mom-finds-son-overdosed-using-call-to-raise-awareness--394027611.html.

37 Brundage, Suzanne C., and Carol Levine. *The Ripple Effect: The Impact of the Opioid Epidemic on Children and Families*. United Hospital Fund, March 2019. https://uhfnyc.org/publications/publication/ripple-effect-opioid-epidemic-children-and-families/

38 Denyse Richter, guest, *It Takes a Village: Addiction Prevention & Recovery on the Seacoast*, podcast series, episode 10, March 16, 2024.

39 Vivian Lefebvre, *It Takes a Village: Addiction Prevention & Recovery on the Seacoast*, podcast series, episode 8, April 15, 2024.

40 GRASP, "About Us." Accessed October 1, 2024. https://grasphelp.org/about-us/.

41 Author interview with Heather Blumenfeld, June 13, 2024.

42 Leslie Jamison, *The Recovering*, Back Bay Books, 2019, 61.

43 McGrath, Michael. "Nancy Reagan's 'Just Say No' Campaign Leaves a Legacy, but What About Today?" *The Guardian*, March 8, 2016. https://www.theguardian.com/society/2016/mar/08/nancy-reagan-drugs-just-say-no-dare-program-opioid-epidemic.

44 Saloner, Brendan, Elizabeth E. McGinty, Leo Beletsky, Ricky Bluthenthal, Chris Beyrer, Michael Botticelli, and Susan G. Sherman. "A Public Health Strategy for the Opioid Crisis." *Public Health Reports* 133, no. 1_suppl (November 2018): 24S-34S.

45 *Boston Sunday Globe,* "What the Drug Reform Movement Missed." April 28, 2024. https://mobileapp.bostonglobe.com/04282024_ff066e74-0170-11ef-9298-47305c20cd48/content.html.

46 New Hampshire Department of Health and Human Services. "Substance Misuse Data Page." Accessed October 1, 2024. https://www.dhhs.nh.gov/programs-services/health-care/substance-misuse-data-page.

47 Quinones, Sam. *The Least of Us: True Tales of America and Hope in the Time of Fentanyl and Meth*. Bloomsbury Publishing, 2021.

48 Beyer, Don. *The Economic Toll of the Opioid Crisis Reached Nearly $1.5 Trillion in 2020*. Joint Economic Committee, 2022.

49 Sherman, Maia. "How Employers Can Support Workers Struggling with Addiction—and Why They Should." *Fortune*. Accessed October 2, 2024. https://fortune.com/longform/drug-addiction-recovery-workplace-support/.

50 Federal Recovery-Ready Workplace Interagency Workgroup. *Recovery-Ready Workplace Toolkit: Guidance and Resources for Private and Public Sector Employers*. 2023. https://www.dol.gov/agencies/eta/RRW-hub/Toolkit.

51 Office of National Drug Control Policy. "Biden-Harris Administration Announces New Actions to Support Recovery-Ready Workplaces and Strengthen Our Economy." *The White House*, November 9, 2023. https://www.whitehouse.gov/ondcp/briefing-room/2023/11/09/biden-harris-administration-announces-new-actions-to-support-recovery-ready-workplaces-and-strengthen-our-economy/.

52 Felitti, Vincent J., Robert F. Anda, Dale Nordenberg, David F. Williamson, Alison M. Spitz, Valerie Edwards, Mary P. Koss, and James S. Marks. "Relationship of Childhood Abuse and Household Dysfunction to Many of the Leading Causes of Death in Adults." *American Journal of Medicine* 14, no. 4 (1998): 245-258.

53 Ibid.

54 McCullough, Larry, guest, *It Takes a Village: Addiction Prevention & Recovery on the Seacoast*, podcast series, episode 2, February 13, 2024.

55   Frederiksen, Lisa. "The Developing Brain & Adverse Childhood Experiences (ACEs)." *PACEs Connection*, 2018. https://www.pacesconnection.com/blog/the-developing-brain-and-adverse -childhood-experiences-aces.

56   Lewis, Elin. "Adverse Childhood Experiences and the Developing Brain." *National Centre for Mental Health*, August 22, 2019. https://www.ncmh.info/2019/08/22/adverse-childhood-experiences -and-the-developing-brain/.

57   PACEs Connection, "ACEs 101: FAQs." Accessed October 2, 2024. https://www.pacesconnection .com/blog/aces-101-faqs.

58   Miller, Ted R., and Nancy N. Carlson. "Adverse Childhood Experiences: Responding to a Cross-Generational Opioid Tragedy." In *Responding to the Opioid Epidemic: A Guide for Public Health Practitioners*, APHA Press, 2024.

59   PACEs, "The Three Realms of ACEs." 2023. https://www.pacesconnection.com/pages /3RealmsACEs.

60   Centers for Disease Control and Prevention. "Risk and Protective Factors for Adverse Child- hood Experiences." Accessed October 2, 2024. https://www.cdc.gov/violenceprevention/aces /riskprotectivefactors.html.

61   Author interview with Lara Merchant, July 31, 2024.

62   Centers for Disease Control and Prevention. "Risk and Protective Factors for Adverse Child- hood Experiences." Accessed October 2, 2024. https://www.cdc.gov/violenceprevention/aces /riskprotectivefactors.html.

63   Author interview with Seth Kaplan, August 23, 2024.

64   Trust for America's Health. *Pain in the Nation: The Epidemics of Alcohol, Drug, and Suicide Deaths.* 2024.

65   Bethell, Christina, Jack Jones, Narangerel Gombojav, Jeffrey Linkenbach, and Robert Sege. "Pos- itive Childhood Experiences and Adult Mental and Relational Health in a Statewide Sample: Associ- ations Across Adverse Childhood Experiences Levels." *JAMA Pediatrics* 173, no. 11 (2019): e193007. https://doi.org/10.1001/jamapediatrics.2019.3007.

66   Bethell, Christina. "Positive Childhood Experiences May Buffer Against Health Effects of Adverse Ones." *All Things Considered*, NPR, 2019.

67   La Charite, J., M. Khan, R. Dudovitz, T. Nuckols, N. Sastry, C. Huang, Y. Lei, and A. Schickedanz. "Specific Domains of Positive Childhood Experiences (PCEs) Associated with Improved Adult Health: A Nationally Representative Study." *SSM—Population Health* 24 (November 11, 2023): 101558.

68   Office of Disease Prevention and Health Promotion. "Social Determinants of Health." *Healthy People 2030*. Accessed October 2, 2024. https://health.gov/healthypeople/priority-areas/social -determinants-health.

69   Block, Peter. *Community: The Structure of Belonging*. Berrett-Koehler Publishers, 2008, 49.

70   Mental Health America. "Connecting with Community." Accessed October 2, 2024. https:// mhanational.org/bipoc/community/connecting-with-community#:~:text=Humans%20are%20 social%20creatures%2C%20meaning,sense%20of%20belonging%20and%20security.

71   National Alliance on Mental Illness. "Building Resilience." Accessed October 2, 2024. https://www. nami.org/Your-Journey/Frontline-Professionals/Public-Safety-Professionals/Building-Resilience.

72   Tamarack Institute. *A Guide for Building a Sustainable and Resilient Collaboration*. n.d.

73 Kaplan, Seth D. *Fragile Neighborhoods: Repairing American Society, One Zip Code at a Time*. Little, Brown Spark, 2023, xiii.

74 Ibid, xvi.

75 Parent, Danielle. "Building Community Resilience After Mass Violence." Workshop presented at the Pinetree Institute 5th Annual Resilience Conference, May 2024.

76 Ibid.

77 Centers for Disease Control and Prevention. "The Role of Trauma-Informed Care in Building Community Resilience." *Public Health Matters Blog*, May 24, 2022. https://blogs.cdc.gov/publichealthmatters /2022/05/trauma-informed/.

78 Center for Health Care Strategies. "What Is Trauma-Informed Care?" Accessed October 2, 2024. https://www.traumainformedcare.chcs.org/what-is-trauma-informed-care/.

79 Molly Louison-Semrow, guest, *It Takes a Village: Addiction & Recovery on the Seacoast* podcast series, episode 1, February 12, 2024.

80 Author interview with Anena Hansen, August 5, 2024.

81 Substance Abuse and Mental Health Services Administration (SAMHSA). *SAMHSA's Working Definition of Recovery*. 2012. https://store.samhsa.gov/sites/default/files/pep12-recdef.pdf.

82 Brundage, Suzanne C., and Carol Levine. *The Ripple Effect: The Impact of the Opioid Epidemic on Children and Families*. United Hospital Fund, 2019.

83 Block, Peter. *The Structure of Belonging*. 2nd ed. Berrett-Koehler Publishers, 2018, xvii–xviii.

84 Kaplan, Seth D. *Fragile Neighborhoods: Repairing American Society, One Zip Code at a Time*. Little, Brown Spark, 2024.

85 Lefebvre, Mark. *A Place in Time: Youth, Community & Baseball*. 2022.

86 Recovery Research Institute. "The Community as the Patient: How to Promote Community Recovery." Accessed October 2, 2024. https://www.recoveryanswers.org/research-post/the-community -as-the-patient-how-to-promote-community-recovery/.

87 "National Peer-Run Training and TA Center for Addiction Recovery Peer Support." *Creating a Recovery-Ready Community*. 2020.

88 Substance Abuse and Mental Health Services Administration (SAMHSA). *Community Engagement: An Essential Component of an Effective and Equitable Substance Use Prevention System*. SAMHSA Publication No. PEP22-06-01-005. Rockville, MD: National Mental Health and Substance Use Policy Laboratory, Substance Abuse and Mental Health Services Administration, 2022.

89 Ashford, R. D., A. M. Brown, R. Ryding, and B. Curtis. "Building Recovery Ready Communities: The Recovery Ready Ecosystem Model and Community Framework." *Addiction Research & Theory* (2019).

90 Faces and Voices of Recovery. "Recovery Capital: Its Role in Sustaining Recovery." Last modified October 8, 2019. https://facesandvoicesofrecovery.org/2019/10/08/recovery-capital-its-role-in -sustaining-recovery/.

91 Webb, Alison Jones, *Recovery Allies: How to Support Addiction Recovery and Build Recovery-Friendly Communities*, North Atlantic Books, 2022, 47.

92 Substance Abuse and Mental Health Services Administration (SAMHSA). *Creating a Recovery-Ready Community*. 2020.

93   Granfield, Robert, and William Cloud. *Coming Clean: Overcoming Addiction without Treatment.* New York: New York University Press, 1999.

94   Faces and Voices of Recovery. "Recovery Capital: Its Role in Sustaining Recovery." Accessed October 2, 2024. https://facesandvoicesofrecovery.org/2019/10/08/recovery-capital-its-role-in-sustaining-recovery/.

95   Elswick, Dr. Alex. "Recovery Capital: Assets Not Abstinence." Presentation, Fletcher Group Webinar, June 6, 2024.

96   Whitesock, David, Jing Zhao, Kristen Goettsch, and Jessica Hanson. "Validating a Survey for Addiction Wellness: The Recovery Capital Index." *South Dakota Medicine* 71, no. 5 (May 2018): 202–212.

97   Author interview with David Whitesock, July 23, 2024.

98   Ibid.

99   Author interview with Lisa Attygalle, August 8, 2024.

100   Tamarack Institute. "The Collective Impact Compendium Tool Series." Accessed October 2, 2024. https://www.tamarackcommunity.ca/interactive-tools/the-collective-impact-compendium -tool-series, 2017.

101   Substance Abuse and Mental Health Services Administration. "Engaging Community Coali- tions to Decrease Opioid Overdose Deaths Practice Guide." Rockville, MD: National Mental Health and Substance Use Policy Laboratory, Substance Abuse and Mental Health Services Administration, 2023, 9.

102   Interview with Ashley Wright, August 21, 2024.

103   Webb, Alison Jones, *Recovery Allies: How to Support Addiction and Build Recovery-Friendly Com- munities,* North Atlantic Books, 2022, 4.

104   ORS Impact and Spark Policy Institute. *When Collective Impact Has an Impact: A Cross-Site Study of 25 Collective Impact Initiatives.* 2018.

105   Molly Louison-Semrow, guest, *It Takes a Village: Addiction & Recovery on the Seacoast* podcast series, episode 1, February 12, 2024.

106   Best, David. *Pathways to Recovery and Desistance.* Policy Press, 2019. Kindle edition, 148.

107   Community Toolbox. "Section 5: Coalition Building 1: Starting a Coalition." Accessed October 2, 2024. https://ctb.ku.edu/en/table-of-contents/assessment/promotion-strategies/start-a-coaltion/main, 2024.

108   Merriam-Webster. "Stigma." Accessed October 2, 2024. https://www.merriam-webster.com/ dictionary/stigma#:~:text=plural%20stigmas%20or%20stigmata%20stig,of%20people%20have%20 about%20something.

109   Jamison, Leslie. *The Recovery: Intoxication and Its Aftermath.* Little, Brown and Company, April 2018, 61.

110   Healthy Androscoggin and the Lewiston-Auburn Area Recovery Collaborative. *Androscoggin County Overdose Prevention and Response Plan.* 2024. (Used with permission).

111   Author interview with Rowan McFadden and Jennifer Edwards, August 28, 2024.

112   Health Androscoggin and the Lewiston Auburn Area Recovery Collaborative. *Androscoggin County Overdose Prevention and Response Plan.* 2024. (Used with permission).

113   State of Maine. "Maine Drug Data Hub." Accessed October 2, 2024. https://mainedrugdata.org/.

114　State of Maine. "Maine Integrated Youth Health Survey." Accessed October 2, 2024. http://www.maine.gov/miyhs/home.

115　Health Androscoggin and the Lewiston Auburn Area Recovery Collaborative. *Androscoggin County Overdose Prevention and Response Plan.* 2024. (Used with permission).

116　Interview with Robin Rieske, July 9, 2024.

117　Interview with Dr. Alex Elswick, June 24, 2024.

118　Webb, Alison Jones, *Recovery Allies: How to Support Addiction and Build Recovery-Friendly Communities,* North Atlantic Books, 2022, p. 3.

119　Author interview with David Whitesock, July 23, 2024.

120　Author interview with Aaron Williams, August 6, 2024.

121　Author interview with Lisa Attygalle, August 8, 2024.

122　Federal Recovery-Ready Interagency Workgroup. *Recovery-Ready Workplace Toolkit.* November 2023, 1.

123　Merriam-Webster. "Friendly." *Merriam-Webster.com Dictionary.* Accessed October 9, 2024. https://www.merriam-webster.com/dictionary/friendly.

124　Merriam-Webster. "Ready." *Merriam-Webster.com Dictionary.* Accessed October 9, 2024. https://www.merriam-webster.com/dictionary/ready.

125　Peer Recovery Center of Excellence. *Increasing Recovery Consciousness: Grounding Systems in Recovery.* 2024.

126　Ibid.

127　Ashford, R. D., Brown, A. M., Ryding, R., and Curtis, B. "Building Recovery Ready Communities: The Recovery Ready Ecosystem Model and Community Framework." *Addiction Research & Theory* 28, no. 1 (2019): 1–11. https://doi.org/10.1080/16066359.2019.1571191.

128　Substance Abuse and Mental Health Services Administration (SAMHSA). *The Recovery-Oriented System of Care (ROSC) Resource Guide.* 2010. https://www.samhsa.gov/sites/default/files/rosc_resource_guide_book.pdf.

129　U.S. Department of Health and Human Services (HHS), Office of the Surgeon General. *Facing Addiction in America: The Surgeon General's Report on Alcohol, Drugs, and Health.* Washington, DC: HHS, November 2016.

130　Best, David. *Pathways to Recovery and Desistance.* Policy Press, 2022. Kindle Edition.

131　Barden, Elizabeth, et al. *092721_TI-ROSC-Toolkit.* National Council for Mental Wellbeing. Accessed October 10, 2024. https://www.thenationalcouncil.org.

132　Ibid.

133　SAMHSA. (2018, October). Trauma and Violence. Retrieved from https://www.samhsa.gov/trauma-violence

134　*DCI Care.* Accessed October 10, 2024. https://www.dcincare.org/.

135　Pinetree Institute, "Building a Recovery Ready Community: A Trauma-Informed Approach," 2024

136　Murphy, Sean. "Alfred to Build Large Detox and Recovery Center, Partner with New Affordable Housing in Sanford." *Spectrum News*, July 16, 2024.

137   Maine Government. "Future of Opioids in Maine." Accessed October 10, 2024. https://www.maine.gov/future/opioids.

138   AdCare Educational Institute. *Strategic Action Plan 2021*. February 2021. https://adcareme.org/wp-content/uploads/2021/02/Strategic-Action-Plan-2021-FINAL.pdf.

139   Interview with Gordon Smith, August 19, 2024.

140   Interview with Leslie Clark, October 2, 2024.

141   Substance Abuse and Mental Health Services Administration (SAMHSA). *A Guide to SAMHSA's Strategic Planning Framework*. 2019.

142   Up for Learning. "Getting to 'Y'." Accessed October 12, 2024. https://www.upforlearning.org/initiatives/getting-to-y/.

143   Longhi, D., and L. Porter. *Community Networks—Building Community Capacity, Reducing Rates of Child and Family Problems: Trends Among Washington State Counties from 1998–2006*. 2009.

144   Search Institute. *The Developmental Relationships Framework*. 2020.

145   Lefebvre, Mark, *A Place in Time: Youth, Community & Baseball*, 2022.

146   National Council for Mental Wellbeing, Center of Excellence for Integrated Health Solutions. "Best Practices: Adolescent Substance Use Disorder Services." 2024. https://www.thenationalcouncil.org/resources/best-practices-adolescent-substance-use-disorder-services/.

147   Eli George, guest, *It Takes a Village: Addiction Prevention & Recovery on the Seacoast* podcast series, episode 13, June 15, 2024.

148   U.S. Department of Health and Human Services (DHHS), Centers for Disease Control and Prevention (CDC), Office of Policy, Performance, and Evaluation. "Framework for Program Evaluation." Accessed October 2, 2024. https://www.cdc.gov/evaluation/steps/step2/index.htm.

149   Lefebvre, Mark. *Lewiston–Auburn Recovery Friendly Workplace Logic Model*. 2022.

150   Molly Louison-Semrow, guest, *It Takes a Village: Addiction & Recovery on the Seacoast* podcast series, episode 1, February 12, 2024.

151   Author interview with David Whitesock, July 23, 2024.

152   Annie Powell, Nyla Christian, Philip Rutherford, Tamara Oyola-Santiago, Tay Saint Amour, Youlim, Song, and Danielle Hornung. "Start with Hope But Don't Stop There." Peer Recovery Center of Excellence, 2024.

153   Equality Community Center. "About Us." Accessed October 19, 2024. https://eccmaine.org/.

154   Sustainability Planning Guide. "Understand the PSAT." Accessed October 12, 2024. https://sustaintool.org/psat/understand/.

155   Tamarack Institute. *Sustainability Self-Assessment Tool*. 2022.

156   CDC National Center for Health Statistics. "U.S. Overdose Deaths Decrease in 2023, First Time Since 2018." 2024.

157   Petras, Hanno, and Zili Sloboda. "17. Opportunities for School-Based Prevention Strategies Responding to the Opioid Epidemic." In *Responding to the Opioid Epidemic: A Guide for Public Health Practitioners*, 2024.

158   Substance Abuse and Mental Health Services Administration (SAMHSA). "Risk and Protective Factors." 2019. https://www.samhsa.gov/sites/default/files/20190718-samhsa-risk-protective-factors.pdf.

159   Ibid.

160 Sarah Fetras, guest, *It Takes a Village: Addiction & Recovery on the Seacoast* podcast series, episode 9, May 19, 2024.

161 Ibid.

162 Ashely Murphy, guest, *It Takes a Village: Addiction & Recovery on the Seacoast* podcast series, episode 14, July 16, 2024.

163 Ringwalt, Chris, DrPH, and Catherine Paton Sandford, MSPH. "Harm Reduction as an Evolving Set of Strategies to Mitigate the Adverse Effects of Illicit Drug Use in the United States." In *Responding to the Opioid Epidemic—A Guide for Public Health Practitioners*, 2024.

164 Liz Beaude, guest, *It Takes a Village: Addiction Prevention & Recovery on the Seacoast* podcast series, episode 12, June 2024.

165 Substance Abuse and Mental Health Services Administration. *Harm Reduction Framework*. Center for Substance Abuse Prevention, Substance Abuse and Mental Health Services Administration, 2023.

166 Harm Reduction Coalition. "About Us." Accessed October 14, 2024. https://harmreduction.org/about-us/.

167 Volunteer New Hampshire. "New Hampshire Recovery Friendly Workplace." Accessed October 14, 2024. https://volunteernh.galaxydigital.com/agency/detail/?agency_id=113935.

168 Wheeler, Paul. "Harm Reduction Clinics in NH Aim to Prevent Overdose Deaths." *Concord Monitor*, May 24, 2024. https://www.concordmonitor.com/Harm-Reduction-Clinics-NH-Prevention-Overdose-Drugs-Concord-NH-54950709.

169 New Hampshire Harm Reduction Collaborative. Accessed October 14, 2024. https://www.nhhrc.org/.

170 Liz Beaude, guest, *It Takes a Village: Addiction Prevention & Recovery on the Seacoast* podcast series, episode 12, June 2024.

171 "Drug Checking Resources: Increase Safety, but Ultimately the Impact Is Uncertain." Recovery Answers. Accessed October 14, 2024. https://www.recoveryanswers.org/research-post/drug-checking-resources-increase-safety-ultimately-impact-is-uncertain/.

172 "Services." Millennium Health. Accessed October 14, 2024. https://www.millenniumhealth.com/services/.

173 Image Safe Supply, Summary of Findings, Canadian Drug Policy Coalition, 2023.

174 Harm Reduction Coalition. "Overview of Supervised Consumption Services in the United States." Accessed October 14, 2024. https://harmreduction.org/issues/supervised-consumption-services/overview-united-states/.

175 Ng, J., Sutherland, C., and Kolber, M. R. "Does Evidence Support Supervised Injection Sites?" *Canadian Family Physician* 63, no. 11 (November 2017): 866. PMID: 29138158; PMCID: PMC5685449.

176 Levengood, T. W., Yoon, G. H., Davoust, M. J., Ogden, S. N., Marshall, B. D. L., Cahill, S. R., and Bazzi, A. R. "Supervised Injection Facilities as Harm Reduction: A Systematic Review." *American Journal of Preventive Medicine* 61, no. 5 (November 2021): 738-749. https://doi.org/10.1016/j.amepre.2021.04.017. Epub July 1, 2021. PMID: 34218964; PMCID: PMC8541900.

177 Brittany Reichmann, guest, *It Takes a Village: Addiction & Recovery on the Seacoast* podcast series, episode 5, April 22, 2024.

178   American Society of Addiction Medicine. *The ASAM National Practice Guideline for the Treatment of Opioid Use Disorder.* American Society of Addiction Medicine, 2020.

179   U.S. Department of Health and Human Services (HHS), Office of the Surgeon General. *Facing Addiction in America: The Surgeon General's Report on Alcohol, Drugs, and Health.* Washington, DC: HHS, November 2016.

180   Substance Abuse and Mental Health Services Administration. *Behavioral Health Treatments and Services.* 2015. Accessed January 25, 2016. http://www.samhsa.gov/treatment.

181   Scutti, Susan. "21 Million Americans Suffer from Addiction. Just 3,000 Physicians Are Specially Trained to Treat Them." *AAMCNEWS.* Accessed September 21, 2024. https://www.aamc.org/news/21-million-americans-suffer-addiction-just-3000-physicians-are-specially-trained-treat-them.

182   Rozansky, Hallie, MD, and Jeffrey Samet, MD, MA, MPH. "Opioid Treatment in Primary Care Settings." In *Responding to the Opioid Epidemic—A Guide for Public Health Practitioners*, 2024.

183   National Academies of Sciences, Engineering, and Medicine. *Medications for Opioid Use Disorder Save Lives.* Washington, DC: The National Academies Press, 2019. https://doi.org/10.17226/25310.

184   Ibid.

185   Clark, H. Westley, MD, JD, MPD, and Matthew Davis. "Medications Used to Treat Opioid Use Disorders." In *Responding to the Opioid Epidemic—A Guide for Public Health Practitioners*, 2024.

186   National Institute on Drug Abuse (NIDA). "How Effective Are Medications to Treat Opioid Use Disorder?" *Research Reports: Medications to Treat Opioid Addiction*, December 3, 2021. Accessed August 26, 2024. https://nida.nih.gov/publications/research-reports/medications-to-treat-opioid-addiction/efficacy-medications-opioid-use-disorder.

187   Substance Abuse and Mental Health Services Administration (SAMHSA). *Substance Use Disorder Treatment for People With Co-Occurring Disorders: Updated 2020.* Rockville, MD: SAMHSA, 2020. Chapter 7, "Treatment Models and Settings for People With Co-Occurring Disorders." Treatment Improvement Protocol (TIP) Series, No. 42. Available from https://www.ncbi.nlm.nih.gov/books/NBK571024/.

188   Substance Abuse and Mental Health Services Administration. *Integrated Treatment for Co-Occurring Disorders: Building Your Program.* DHHS Pub. No. SMA-08-4366. Rockville, MD: Center for Mental Health Services, Substance Abuse and Mental Health Services Administration, U.S. Department of Health and Human Services, 2009.

189   "Co-Occurring Disorder." Recovery Research Institute. Accessed October 15, 2024. https://www.recoveryanswers.org/resource/co-occurring-disorders/.

190   Center for Substance Abuse Treatment. *A Guide to Substance Abuse Services for Primary Care Clinicians.* Rockville, MD: Substance Abuse and Mental Health Services Administration, 1997. (Treatment Improvement Protocol [TIP] Series, No. 24.) Chapter 5—Specialized Substance Abuse Treatment Programs. Available from: https://www.ncbi.nlm.nih.gov/books/NBK64815/.

191   Interview with Laura Pratt, September 25, 2024.

192   All Rise. "About Treatment Courts." Accessed October 19, 2024. https://allrise.org/about/treatment-courts/.

193   Ibid.

194   Tina Nadeau, guest, *It Takes a Village: Addiction & Recovery on the Seacoast* podcast series, episode 7, 2024.

195   Cheryll Andrews, guest, *It Takes a Village: Addiction & Recovery on the Seacoast* podcast series, episode 17, November 17, 2024.

196   Maine Recovery Residences. "Maine Recovery Residences." Accessed October 15, 2024. https://www.mainerecoveryresidences.com/.

197   National Alliance for Recovery Residences. "Standards for Recovery Residences." Accessed October 15, 2024. https://narronline.org/standards/#types-of-recovery-residences.

198   Cheryll Andrews, guest, *It Takes a Village: Addiction & Recovery on the Seacoast* podcast series, episode 17, November 17, 2024.

199   Jules Johnson, guest, *It Takes a Village: Addiction & Recovery on the Seacoast* podcast series, episode 15, August 15, 2024.

200   Peer Recovery Center of Excellence. "RCO Capacity Building." Accessed October 16, 2024. https://peerrecoverynow.org/focus-areas/rco-capacity-building/.

201   Faces and Voices of Recovery. "National Standards for Recovery Community Organizations." Accessed October 16, 2024. https://facesandvoicesofrecovery.org/resource/national-standards-for-recovery-community-organizations/.

202   "Hope for New Hampshire Recovery Joins Forces with National Non-Profit to Expand Services." *Manchester Ink Link*, Accessed October 16, 2024. https://manchester.inklink.news/hope-nh-joins-forces-national-non-profit-expand-services/.

203   "The RECOVER Project—About Us." Accessed October 16, 2024. https://recoverproject.org/about/.

204   "SOS Recovery Community Organization." Accessed October 16, 2024. https://sosrco.org/.

205   "Granite Pathways." Accessed October 16, 2024. https://granitepathwaysnh.org/.

206   Portland Recovery Community Center. "Portland Recovery." Accessed October 16, 2024. https://portlandrecovery.org/.

207   Interview with Leslie Clark, October 2, 2024.

208   Ibid.

209   Federal Recovery-Ready Workplace Interagency Workgroup. "Recovery-Ready Workplace Toolkit: Guidance and Resources for Private and Public Sector Employers." 2023. www.dol.gov/agencies/eta/RRW-hub/Toolkit

210   Recovery Friendly Workplace. "Home." Accessed October 2, 2024. https://www.recoveryfriendlyworkplace.com/.

211   Staatz, Christine, Lauren Blyler, Jake Bodenlos, Kerrie Mack, and Ivan Gutierrez. National Health Emergency Grants to Address the Opioid Crisis: Implementation Study Final Report. 2021.

212   Walton M.T., Hall M.T. "The Effects of Employment Interventions on Addiction Treatment Outcomes: A Review of the Literature." *Journal of Social Work Practice in the Addictions.* 2016;16(4):358-384

213   Pinetree Institute: Recovery Friendly Workplace Report to Maine Health Access Foundation, June 2022.

214   Ibid.

215   Colleen Staatz, Jillian Berk, Crystal Blyler, Katie Bodenios, Melissa Mack, and Ivette Gutierrez, National Health Emergency Grants to Address the Opioid Crisis: Implementation Study Final Report, 2021.

216   https://granitepathwaysnh.org/job-launch-2/.

217   https://workingfields.com/employers.php.

218   Author interview with Chelsea Bardot Lewis, September 13, 2024.

219   Federal Recovery-Ready Workplace Interagency Workgroup. Recovery-Ready Workplace Tool-kit: Guidance and Resources for Private and Public Sector Employers. 2023. www.dol.gov/agencies/eta/RRW-hub/Toolkit

220   Samantha Lewandowski and Jeanne Venuti, guests, *It Takes a Village: Addiction & Recovery on the Seacoast* podcast series, episode 18, November, 2024.

221   Ibid.

222   Interview with Eliza Zarka, October 22, 2024.

223   Author interview with Brittany Reichmann, September 12, 2024.

224   La Vigne, Nancy, Elizabeth Davies, Tobi Palmer, and Robin Halberstadt. *Release Planning for Successful Reentry: A Guide for Corrections, Service Providers, and Community Groups.* Urban Institute Justice Policy Center, 2008.

225   Beck, Allen, Marcus Berzofsky, Rachel Caspar, and Christopher Krebs. *Sexual Victimization in Prisons and Jails Reported by Inmates, 2011-12: National Inmate Survey, 2011-12.* U.S. Department of Justice, 2013.

226   Substance Abuse and Mental Health Services Administration. *Guidelines for Successful Transition of People with Mental or Substance Use Disorders from Jail and Prison: Implementation Guide.* 2017.

227   Maine Reentry Network (MERN). *Reentry Resource Guide.* 2021.

228   Interview with Bruce Noddin, September 25, 2024.

229   Ratcliff, Michael, Charlynn Burd, Kelly Holder, and Alison Fields. "Defining Rural at the U.S. Census Bureau." December 2016.

230   University of Vermont Center on Rural Addiction (May 2022). *Data Report—Maine Baseline Needs Assessment: Rural Practitioners and Stakeholders.* Accessed September, 30, 2024. https://www.uvmcora.org/wp-content/uploads/2022/05/Maine-BNA-Rural-Practitioners-and-Stakeholders-Report-May-2022.pdf.

231   University of Vermont Center on Rural Addiction (April 2024). *Qualitative Data Brief—Perspectives on Opioid Use Disorder Treatment Access and Engagement from Rural Family Members and People in Treatment.* Accessed September 30, 2024. https://www.uvmcora.org/wp-content/uploads/2024/12/SumBriefReport_CORA_family_April-2024_FINAL-s.pdf.

232   Fletcher Group. *How to Handle NIMBYism.* Fletcher Group RCOE Guide. Accessed via Chrome extension. https://www.fletchergroup.org/wp-content/uploads/2022/03/FLETCHER-GROUP-RCOE-GUIDE-HOW-TO-HANDLE-NIMBYism.pdf.

233   City of Portsmouth Community Development Department. *Portsmouth in the Present.* 2012.

234   New Hampshire Employment Security. "Portsmouth Community Profile." Accessed October 16, 2024. https://www.nhes.nh.gov/elmi/products/cp/profiles-htm/portsmouth.htm.

235   Zillow. "70 Meadow Rd, Portsmouth, NH 03801." Accessed October 16, 2024. https://www.zillow.com/homedetails/70-Meadow-Rd-Portsmouth-NH-03801/95360320_zpid/.

236   Meier, A., Moore, S. K., Saunders, E. C., McLeman, B., Metcalf, S. A., Auty, S., Walsh, O., and Marsch, L. A. "Understanding the Increase in Opioid Overdoses in New Hampshire: A Rapid Epidemiologic Assessment." *Drug and Alcohol Dependence* 209 (2020): 107893. https://doi.org /10.1016/j.drugalcdep.2020.107893.

237   "Why New Hampshire Has One of the Highest Rates of Opioid-Related Deaths." *U.S. News & World Report,* June 28, 2017. https://www.usnews.com/news/best-states/articles/2017-06-28 /why-new-hampshire-has-one-of-the-highest-rates-of-opioid-related-deaths.

238   "NH Drug Monitoring Initiative." *NH Information & Analysis Center,* October 2020 Report, November 2020.

239   University of New Hampshire Institute for Health Policy and Practice and Foundation for Seacoast Health, *Seacoast-Area Health Assessments Review,* 2023.

240   "The Doorway." *New Hampshire Department of Health and Human Services.* Accessed October 16, 2024. https://www.thedoorway.nh.gov/.

241   Nadeau, Honorable Tina, guest, *It Takes A Village: Addiction Prevention & Recovery on the Seacoast* podcast series, episode 7, April 2, 2024.

242   Larry McCullough, guest, *It Takes a Village: Addiction & Recovery on the Seacoast* podcast series, episode 1, January 12, 2024.

243   New Hampshire Department of Health and Human Services. *Division for Behavioral Health: Delivery System and Market Impact Review 2021 Overview.* Accessed October 20, 2024. https://www. dhhs.nh.gov/sites/g/files/ehbemt476/files/documents2/dmi-2021overview.pdf.

244   Cliff Lazenby, guest, *It Takes a Village: Addiction & Recovery on the Seacoast* podcast series, episode 16, September 15, 2024.

245   WSCA 106.1 FM. *It Takes a Village: Addiction & Recovery on the Seacoast.* Accessed October 20, 2024. https://wscafm.org/it-takes-a-village-addiction-prevention-recovery-on-the-seacoast/.

246   Molly Louison-Semrow, guest, *It Takes a Village: Addiction & Recovery on the Seacoast* podcast series, episode 1, February 12, 2024.

INDEX

York County, Maine, 83–84
youth. *See also* ACEs (adverse childhood experiences); childhood trauma; positive childhood experiences (PCEs)
  Alternative Peer Group, 136
  anxiety, 91, 107
  community ecosystems for, 30
  depression and, 91
  developmental relationships, 89–90, 115
  health and wellness, 88–91, 107
  mental health, 90–91, 107–109
  prevention capacity, 89–91
  prevention strategies for, 106, 174–175
  protective factors, 25–26, 89, 106
  residential treatment, 108
  resilience, 25, 29–30
  restorative justice, 107, 109
  at-risk, 108–109
  risk factors, 106
  suicide risk, 40, 109
trauma-informed services, 107–109
youth and family programming, 106–109

Z

Zadravec, Stephen, 170, 183
Zarka, Eliza, 149

ABOUT THE AUTHOR

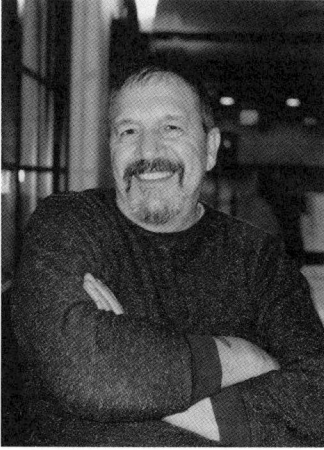

MARK LEFEBVRE is the founder and was statewide director for the Maine Recovery Friendly Workplace (RFW) program, where he focused on building statewide capacity to recruit, train and support Maine businesses as Recovery Friendly Workplaces. In his prior role as the Pinetree Director of Community Engagement, Mark was responsible for the development of Recovery-Ready Communities in the Seacoast of New Hampshire and Southern Maine.

Before joining the Pinetree Institute, Mark served as program director for the NH Works for Recovery program at Southern NH Services. He oversaw outreach and delivery of employment and training services to individuals and families affected by the New Hampshire opioid crisis and helped launch New Hampshire's Recovery Friendly Workplace program. Previously, he had served on New Hampshire Governor Sununu's Commission as a member of both the Prevention and Recovery Task Forces.

Mark Lefebvre is a person in long-term recovery from addiction and is the author of the book *A Place in Time: Youth, Community & Baseball*, a consultant, a radio DJ, and a podcast producer. Mark and his wife Vivian are co-founders of Safe Harbor Recovery Center in Portsmouth, New Hampshire, and live on the Seacoast of New Hampshire with their yellow lab mix rescue dog, Layla.